Studies in the Psychosocial

Studies in the Psychosocial seeks to investigate the ways in which psychic and social processes demand to be understood as always implicated in each other, as mutually constitutive, co-produced, or abstracted levels of a single dialectical process. As such it can be understood as an interdisciplinary field in search of transdisciplinary objects of knowledge. Studies in the Psychosocial is also distinguished by its emphasis on affect, the irrational and unconscious processes, often, but not necessarily, understood psychoanalytically. Studies in the Psychosocial aims to foster the development of this field by publishing high quality and innovative monographs and edited collections. The series welcomes submissions from a range of theoretical perspectives and disciplinary orientations, including sociology, social and critical psychology, political science, postcolonial studies, feminist studies, queer studies, management and organization studies, cultural and media studies and psychoanalysis. However, in keeping with the inter- or transdisciplinary character of psychosocial analysis, books in the series will generally pass beyond their points of origin to generate concepts, understandings and forms of investigation that are distinctively psychosocial in character.

Ana C. Minozzo

# Anxiety as Vibration

## A Psychosocial Cartography

palgrave
macmillan

Ana C. Minozzo
Psychosocial and Psychoanalytic Studies
University of Essex
Colchester, UK

ISSN 2662-2629 ISSN 2662-2637 (electronic)
Studies in the Psychosocial
ISBN 978-3-031-62855-9 ISBN 978-3-031-62856-6 (eBook)
https://doi.org/10.1007/978-3-031-62856-6



Cover illustration: amtitus/ Getty Images

This Palgrave Macmillan imprint is published by the registered company Springer Nature Switzerland AG.
The registered company address is: Gewerbestrasse 11, 6330 Cham, Switzerland

Paper in this product is recyclable.

*To all feminists, anxious or not, past, present and future.*

# Acknowledgements

This book has materialised as a co-poetic effort and as a result of acts of generosity, love and friendship.

I am immensely grateful for the contributions of Stephen Frosh, Rosi Braidotti, Magarita Palacios, Leticia Sabsay, Angie Voela, Léa Silveira, Raluca Soreanu and all colleagues from the former Department of Psychosocial Studies at Birkbeck, University of London. Grateful to Dorothée Bonnigal-Katz, Kati Gray and colleagues of the Psychosis Therapy Project who keep the ethics of psychoanalysis alive, every day. I am also grateful for having encountered Berjanet Jazani and for the transformative work done together. Thankful to my feminist friends of GEPEF, peers from The Site for Contemporary Psychoanalysis, friends made during my time at CFAR and our international network of analysts, researchers and unconscious-enthusiasts. I am grateful for the tremendous incentive of my colleagues from FREEPSY, at the University of Essex, and our comrades in the UK, Europe, Latin America and beyond.

This book is being published as an Open Access resource only thanks to the tremendous institutional support of the University of Essex. Special thanks to Hannah Crago and Sean Anderson. Thanks to Beth Farrow, at Palgrave; Tikoji Rao, at Springer Nature, and the board of editors of the Studies in the Psychosocial series.

# About the Book

This book offers an in depth and radical survey of the status of anxiety in our times. By combining a multidisciplinary approach to this ubiquitous affect, the book examines the troubles of contemporary diagnoses and points out to possibilities of forging a creative clinic. The book takes a feminist, non-Oedipal stance towards psychoanalytic texts, and invites art theory, medical humanities and philosophy for a conversation that answers the question: *What can anxiety do?*

Anxiety, for Lacan, is an affect that sits between desire and *jouissance*; it is an encounter with the Real that mobilises or squeezes the subject between a Symbolically wrapped delineation of oneself, which hangs by a thread once the Imaginary fantasy of consistency fails, and the vastness and abyss that extend beyond oneself, the Real. Interestingly, anxiety is shunted out of the DSM-III (Diagnostic and Statistical Manual of Mental Disorders) when the biologistic and pharmaceutical paradigms of psychiatry gain strength over psychoanalysis after the 1970s, only to return as a companion to a biomedicalised depression. The affect of anxiety is, thus, pathologised and locked into a state of estrangement, without, however, opening up to possible new ways of living, revealing a mode of affective alienation Deleuze calls a 'dividualisation'.

In this book we will explore the possibilities of an encounter with the Real as a sphere of excessive affect in psychoanalysis, calling this meeting a vibration. Anchoring our enquiry on the art practice of Lygia Clark, the book utilises vibration as a conceptual artifice when thinking of affects beyond an Oedipal frame, beyond ego-to-ego relations and a short-circuit of individualised bodily *jouissance*. Or, as Clark named it, beyond the 'Plane' into where lies the 'full-void'. We ask: What can psychoanalysis do that addresses the battles of psychic suffering and, at the same time, decentres the modern humanist subject, opening possibilities for the creation of new ways of living, of new worlds? Anxiety is the affect we work with in the search for a critique of the dividualising residues in psychoanalysis of the Freudian and Lacanian orientation, moving towards an entangled, situated and creative clinic, shifting from the paradigm of interpretation to that of *co-poiesis*.

## Chapter 1: Introduction: Anxiety

In the introduction, I set the psychosocial scope of this book and situate the reader into the urgency of reframing the clinic of anxiety. The key concepts worked in the book such as vibration, co-poiesis and the Real are first introduced.

## Chapter 2: The Full-Void of Anxiety

This chapter elaborates the notion of a 'full-void' in dialogue with the art practice of Lygia Clark. Key questions about the limits of psychoanalytic classic interpretations are posed, compelling the reader to be curious about the method of co-poiesis.

## Chapter 3: The Production of Anxiety

This chapter offers a critical survey of the history of diagnosing and treating anxiety across the last century. Under a medical humanities frame, we set out the political and clinical issues of diagnosing anxiety and the grammar offered to suffering in contemporary times

## Chapter 4: Abysses and Horizons: Why Psychoanalysis?

Questioning the possibilities of introducing the unconscious in the understanding of anxiety, this chapter works with a philosophical and feminist critique to what is considered normal and pathological.

## Chapter 5: Libidinal Excesses

This chapter offers a unique and complete survey of Freud's shifting ideas on anxiety. By detailing the formation of his thought on the topic, we are able to map the different moments of relying on the Oedipal metaphor and working with anxiety metapsychologically. The chapter covers the nineteenth century letters until his last published pieces.

## Chapter 6: Edging the Real

This chapter traces a detailed and yet accessible summary of Lacan's theories, zooming into his works on anxiety. From the stance of a psychosocial clinic, we cover his theories from the first seminar until his later seminars. The chapter offers a unique overview of Lacan's later theories in relation to anxiety.

## Chapter 7: Vibrating the Full-Void

This chapter invites the reader into a creative questioning of the limits of Freudian and Lacanian theories when it comes to the clinic of anxiety. Thinking with Spinoza and Rosi Braidotti, as well as the artist Lygia Clark, we open space to the possibilities of anxiety as an affect.

## Chapter 8: The Trail of Vibration

This chapter introduces the read in depth to the work of Deleuze and Guattari. Addressing the psychosocial shortcomings of Freud and Lacan, we explore their contributions under the concept of vibration. This chapter proposes a unique overview of what would be a Guattarian theory of anxiety.

## Chapter 9: Conclusion: Co-Poiesis on the Couch

In conclusion, we mark the edges of psychoanalytic theory and practice and argue for a creative clinic of anxiety in dialogue with psychosocial texts and interventions.

# Praise for *Anxiety as Vibration*

"This book vibrates with hope, tracking traditional psychoanalytic arguments about anxiety in a marvellously clear way, and opening up possibilities in cultural and clinical practice for a bodily engagement with the theories of subjectivity that shape us, that frame contemporary commonsense. Ana Minozzo gives us exposition, argument and alternative, a rare achievement, ground-breaking and shaking us to think anew about anxiety and do something different with it."

—Ian Parker, psychoanalyst, Honorary Professor of Education, *University of Manchester, UK*

"Minozzo's *Anxiety as Vibration* is a terrific and impressive read: a lively and scholarly cross-disciplinary work, it dissects anxiety in its pharmaceutical logics, its psychoanalytic understandings, and its artistic potential, and the resulting work amounts to an energetic exploration of anxiety as an altogether more fascinating state than we might usually allow. I thoroughly enjoyed it and cannot recommend it enough."

—Katherine Angel, writer, author of *Tomorrow Sex Will be Good Again*

"In *Anxiety as Vibration*, Ana Minozzo transgresses the limits of classic psychoanalytic practice and theory providing a complex and contemporary concept of anxiety. It is described both as central figure of psycho-estrangement and as a possible focus of resistance and entanglement. In this sense, Minozzo asks not only what can be done to anxiety but also points towards Spinozian answers of 'what anxiety can do'. On the basis of a transversal reading of the history and conceptuality of anxiety, the book offers a feminist perspective on Freud and Lacan. Against individualist and normalizing concepts of wellbeing and pathology it arrives at the necessity of reinventing psychoanalysis, in an aberrant clinic of anxiety and with the help of relational concepts like co-poiesis, sinthôme, and vibration."

—Gerald Raunig, philosopher, author of *Making Multiplicity*

"In this startlingly creative work, Ana Minozzo weaves together artistic, clinical and theoretical modes of enquiry to demonstrate the paradoxical yet essential value of anxiety for the modern, entangled subject. Defying psychoanalytic orthodoxies, Minozzo upends individualising methods of managing suffering through her invention of a 'vibrational' clinical practice. Forget intoxication—read this book and feel the vibration!"

—Jordan Osserman, *University of Essex, UK*,
author of *Circumcision on the Couch*

# Contents

# About the Author

**Ana C. Minozzo** is a psychoanalyst and researcher based in London, UK, and originally from Brazil. She has gained a PhD in Psychosocial Studies from Birkbeck, University of London, and has a background of teaching and collaborating with international projects and institutions of psychoanalysis and the arts. Ana is currently a Postdoctoral Researcher in Psychosocial Studies at the University of Essex, UK, and part of the FREEPSY collective research on the legacies of free psychoanalytic clinics. Her clinical experience ranges from working in several community-based mental health services, including working with children, the LGBTQI+ community, refugees and those seeking asylum to working with Latin American women and migrants. She is a member of The Site for Contemporary Psychoanalysis and a collaborator of the Psychosis Therapy Project, both in London, UK. Ana has contributed to a number of books such as *Psicanálise e esquizoanálise: Diferença e Composição* (2022), São Paulo, n-1 edições; *The Palgrave Handbook of Psychosocial Studies.* ed. Frosh, S.; Vyrgioti, M. and Walsh, J. (2022–2023) London: Palgrave Macmillan; *Freud e o Patriarcado* (2020) Sao Paulo, Hedra; and *New Voices in Psychosocial Studies.* ed. Frosh, S. (2019) London: Palgrave Macmillan. This is her first monograph.

# 1

# Introduction: Anxiety

We often hear that we, as society, have never been so anxious. If that's so, then what could we do with all this anxiety? Is it possible to consider that we can experience it, traverse it, towards some sort of emancipation rather than being further subjugated, medicalised or simply paralysed by our anxiety?

This is a psychosocial cartography anxiety which takes you, reader, for a long and deep walk towards a creative clinic of this puzzling affect—our site, destiny and point of departure all at once. Accompanying us are several psychosocial scholars, psychoanalysts and feminists past and present. In our travels, these disciplines and traditions of scholarship will also be questioned in light of the forms of subjective and social alienation they produce and reproduce. In this sense, anxiety matters on the couch but also outside of it. If you are a clinician, researcher, artist or activist, this is an invitation of thinking-together.

The ubiquitous anxious sensation of dread, breathlessness, paralysation and panic has been at the centre of debates in psychiatry, psychology, psychoanalysis and the target of wellness rituals and advice over the last century. Measured by governments as a sign of populational lack of well-being, medicated *en masse* in primary care and heard as a common complaint of those arriving at a psychoanalytic couch—often after having


A. C. Minozzo, *Anxiety as Vibration*, Studies in the Psychosocial,
https://doi.org/10.1007/978-3-031-62856-6_1

tried other methods and therapies to ease their suffering—anxiety has been called a 'silent epidemic' affecting a fifth of the population in places such as the United States and the United Kingdom (Cooke, 2013; Bandelow & Michaelis, 2015).

In psychoanalysis, since Freud, anxiety is curiously not something to get rid of so fast, or the problem itself. Rather, it is an affect integral to psychic experience that functions as a signal of a threat to the ego (Freud, 1917, 1926). Being so, anxiety is considered to be a 'compass' in the mapping of an analytic treatment (Miller, 2007). Some clinical approaches within psychiatry and the psychologies, such as Positive Psychology, and even psychoanalytic orientations from a British and North-American tradition, find value in strengthening one's ego defences against the hurricane that anxiety may feel like. In the Freudian and Lacanian orientations, broadly speaking, however, making the ego more malleable, capable of riding the sweeping waves from the unconscious that become apparent in anxiety, is the direction of the treatment in which anxiety is not a stranger to the self; instead, it is entangled in the life of the subject, in their abysses and horizons.

In this book, I take you for a cartographic-trip to the possible 'full-void' of anxiety, arguing that psychoanalysis not only offers valuable insights into what one's anxiety is all about as it also opens possibilities for the constructions of new modes of living departing from the rupture to the self that characterises the experience of anxiety. My writing here, which comes as a result of an extensive research combined with years of clinical practice privately and in community projects, makes the point that psychoanalysis, when (and if) read through non-Oedipal lenses, informs not only what can be done to anxiety but also points towards answers of 'what anxiety can do'.

In looking for the clues to the possibilities of anxiety as an affect, I will trace a route into a creative clinic, one that holds on to what I call psychoanalytic 'vibrational moments' where the affect of anxiety takes the subject away from an abyss-within into a horizon-beyond oneself. In doing so, I explore the possibilities of 'being' and 'becomings' for psychoanalysis by thinking through the potentialities of rupture in the psychoanalytic clinic, and also, what to do with it: interpret rupture within structural frames or mobilise it into novel and collective ways of being, assembling it through the technique of *co-poiesis*, as we learn holding hands with the late-Brazilian artist Lygia Clark and inspiring thinkers such as Félix Guattari and Rosi Braidotti, all of whom have shaken psychoanalytic pillars in their own way. Such balance is a subtle and yet serious political matter that crosses feminist, ecological and decolonial demands and critiques to the clinical and epistemological pillars of analytic praxis. At the same time, it speaks to the mundane, here-and-now, experiences of anxiety we are understood to be all immersed in.

In this psychosocial cartography, I set psychoanalysis and its potential approach to anxiety as resting between a 'dividualising' alienating modulation of affect—which relies on the Oedipal paradigm of domination and castration—and the plane of immanence Lygia Clark (1994) calls a 'full-void', which vibrates through the subject what extends beyond oneself as an ethics of multiplicity and togetherness (Deleuze, 1992; Braidotti, 1994, 2006). Exploring the troubles and the promises of both a 'dividualising' and a 'vibrational' model of psy, I search for the psychoanalytic unconscious in its moment of excess, rupture and too-muchness that characterises anxiety—or, an anxiety as vibration, in search of a psychosocial creative clinic. This clinic is a clinic where other worlds are possible and unfold in the complicated threshold of necessity and possibility—or what is, was and what could be.

## References

Bandelow, B., & Michaelis, S. (2015). Epidemiology of Anxiety Disorders in the 21st century. *Dialogues in Clinical Neuroscience, 17*(3), 327–335.

Braidotti, R. (1994). *Nomadic Subjects: Embodiment and Sexual Difference in Contemporary Feminist Theory*. Columbia University Press.

Braidotti, R. (2006). *Transpositions: On Nomadic ethics*. Polity Press.

Clark, L. (1994). Nostalgia of the Body. *October, 69*(Summer), 85–109.

Cooke, R. (2013, September 15). Living with Anxiety: Britain's Silent Epidemic. *The Guardian*. Sunday. [Online]. https://www.theguardian.com/society/2013/sep/15/anxiety-epidemic-gripping-britain

Deleuze, G. (1992). Postscript on Societies of Control. *October, 59*, 3–7.

Freud, S. (1917). Introductory Lectures on Psycho-Analysis. In *The Standard Edition of the Complete Psychological Works of Sigmund Freud, Volume XVI (1916–1917): Introductory Lectures on Psycho-Analysis (Part III)* (pp. 241–463). The Hogarth Press and the Institute of Psychoanalysis.

Freud, S. (1926). Inhibitions, Symptoms and Anxiety. In *The Standard Edition of the Complete Psychological Works of Sigmund Freud, Volume XX (1925–1926): An Autobiographical Study, Inhibitions, Symptoms and Anxiety, The Question of Lay Analysis and Other Works* (pp. 75–176). The Hogarth Press and the Institute of Psychoanalysis.

Miller, J. A. (2007). *La angustia—Introducción al Seminario X de Jacques Lacan*. Gredos.

# 2

# The Full-Void of Anxiety

*The 'full-void' contains all potentialities*
—Lygia Clark

Clinicians can often benefit from some more creativity, from stretching our imaginative capacity beyond the tenets of classic texts. When welcoming a patient expressing their struggles with anxiety—what we call a 'complaint', in psychoanalysis—we are invited to listen and pay attention to different things: repetitions, patterns, structures, functions or escapes. Whilst any ethical listener in our field is attentive to singularity, or simply attuned to avoiding making generalised interpretations and putting others in a box, formative myths of the unconscious are frequent guests in the way analysts think or speak. Oedipus, castration, family, gender and sex identifications. What will become clearer as we move along in this book is that such anchors are not without consequence and there are benefits, clinically and politically, about stretching clinical interventions psychosocially.

Anxiety complaints are commonly bodily complaints: my heart, my stomach, my hands. I sweat. I shake. I wake up at night. I stop. Lygia


A. C. Minozzo, *Anxiety as Vibration*, Studies in the Psychosocial,
https://doi.org/10.1007/978-3-031-62856-6_2

Clark, as an artist of 'borders', found a way of listening to the body in her inventive and unorthodox art/therapy practice. For this reason, as we will see in what follows, there is value in thinking about her experimentation with that which anxiety captures in our daily phenomenological experience of it: our bodies. Her practice will ground our imagination in this abstract and fugitive path within the guts of classic texts by Freud, Lacan, Deleuze and Guattari that feature in this book, helping us to arrive there with more (feminist) creativity.

In order to hold onto the crossroads of anxiety itself, paralysing yet moving, I suggest we travel far from classic epidemiologic or clinical discussions and, before going there, embark on this psychosocial cartography of anxiety to discover together the idea of the 'full-void'—which we will pack in our suitcase in this first moment.

## Moving Beyond the Limits of the Plane

A prominent artist of her time and to this day one of the biggest names in Brazilian art, my compatriot Lygia Clark was very influenced by her experience in psychoanalysis as a patient. Working during the Brazilian military dictatorship that lasted from the 1960s to the 1980s, and witnessing the very early announcement of neoliberal politics in Europe, the United States and Latin America, she developed, in the later stage of her prolific career, a practice marked by what she named an 'abandonment of the art world'. Clark is notable for her singular practice involving the body: her body, the body of viewers and the possibilities of bodies. Specifically, hers was a practice called 'Nostalgia of the Body', which she defined as a process of corporeal fragmentation towards and through the process of reconstructing the body as a 'collective body' (Rivera, 2013). This trajectory of leaving the art world and embarking on a psychotherapeutic proposition can be followed in her essay 'Nostalgia of the Body', published posthumously in 1994 in the *October* journal, which we will examine together.

In a passage entitled 'Death of a Plane', Clark qualifies the discontent with the elementary form of artistic practice—the 'plane', or the square, the canvas—that led her to embark on a journey beyond such a 'false idea of reality' projected by humanity within this limiting frame:

> The plane is a concept created by humanity to serve practical ends: that of satisfying its need for balance [...]. The plane arbitrarily marks off the limits of a space giving humanity an entirely false and rational idea of its own reality [...]. It's also the reason why people have projected their transcendent part outward and given it the name of God. In this way the problem of their own existence is raised in inventing the mirror of their own spirituality [...]. But the plane is dead. The philosophical conception that humanity projected onto it no longer satisfies—no more than does the idea of an external God persist. In becoming aware that it is a matter of an internal poetry of the self that is projected into the exterior it is understood at the same time that this poetry must be reintegrated as an indivisible part of the individual. (Clark, 1994, p. 96)

The plane is charged with her cosmological dissatisfaction with the need for an 'external God' as an obstacle to an 'internal poetry' that pertains to the self. In this sense, I suggest one could interpret the 'plane' as what Lacanian psychoanalysis calls the net of signifiers anchored in an Imaginary relation to language and culture that is always dependent on a transcendental Other, as Lacan calls it, to have any consistency. Perhaps, if we may, the same thing universalising coloniality has deemed to be the 'World' of the 'Human', all in capitals. Following this logic, Clark's move towards a practice that liberates this 'internal poetry' is akin to an endeavour of tracing an ontological possibility that gives space for an immanence in desire that is not reliant on the relationship with the Other and the inscribed Oedipal Law-of-the-Father, as psychoanalysis demands and we will consider together, but to several 'others' in space, tracing a different ecological cartography to the subject. This is Clark's feminist twist, as I quite like to think of it: against universals and proposing an ethics of multiplicity. Her endeavour is exactly of the order I wish to find conditions for in the psychoanalytic clinic of anxiety, and this will require, from us, some creativity and imagination too. As we dive into her world, can we hold onto the possibilities and necessities of the 'many', rather than the 'one'?

* * *

Practicing art since 1947, when she moved to Rio de Janeiro from her native Minas Gerais, Lygia Clark's most significant breakthrough in the artistic scene came with the publication of the *Neo-Concrete Manifesto*, in 1959. Her association with the Neo-concrete group and their push towards sensibility over the rationality of Concretism already carry something of her travel 'beyond the Plane', which is present in their discontentment with the standardised practices of artists and curators around her. Clark's bolder 'killing of the Plane' starts in the 1960s, in her departure from the formalist geometrical painting and sculpture that ignited her career, and in the development of works such as *Bichos* and *Caminhando* (1963–1964), which called the viewer to a closer contact with the artworks, touching and participating. *Bichos*, a series of multidimensional metallic forms joined by hinges, invites the spectator to be co-author of the piece by moving it. In this work we see a dual interaction of entities (human/aluminium structure or spectator/artist) brought to the same level by movement. Or, we could say, in this early interactive piece we see a 'levelling of the Plane', before Clark really moves into perforating it.

In *Caminhando*, a Möbius strip appears as the topological resource to bring her flight beyond the limits of the plane to the debate between in/out, where not only the relation between subject/object was questioned but the actual reality of 'being in space'. In this work, for the first time in her career, the 'act' thus gains more importance over the 'object'. The piece moves towards a rupture, as each repetition tightens and slows the movement of scissors over paper. As I see it, this movement towards rupture via a repetition, present in this piece, is also her move beyond the 'plane'. The action of *Caminhando* offers a metaphor of the psychoanalytic fantasy, or of the Death Drive, which implies a constant repetition, moving without leaving the same spot—this being Lacan's view that all 'drives' operate as a repetitive 'death drive' (Lacan, 1966, p. 848), clearly leaving us, in times of eco-feminist catastrophes, thirsty for some rays of Life. In this sense, Clark's *Caminhando* is a subversion of the status of the subject, which in her work is not confined to the tragic repetition of the same but is moving towards a rupture. The subjective crisis in such metaphoric gesture is, as Tania Rivera (2008) sees it, a subjective awakening upon the exit of specular alienation. From then onwards, objects would not mean the same to Clark (limited to the status of 'art objects'), and would no longer represent the limiting spatial cut of the 'plane'. From

*Caminhando* until her death, in 1988, "the object would lose its *thingness* to become, once more, a field of living forces that affect, and are affected, by the world, promoting a continuous process of differentiation of subjective and objective realities" (Rolnik, 2013a, p. 76; 2013b). Her work thus crosses the plane and embarks on a journey through the body and affect.

## Bodies of/at Work

While Clark 'kills the plane' and slowly 'abandons the art world', her surroundings shift dramatically. On a very concrete level, the Brazilian Military coup of March 1964 inaugurated two decades of dictatorship in Brazil—a period of repressive censorship and violence that also loomed over other Latin American countries. In the art world, censorship was explicit. Just like at universities, the artistic environment was severely sabotaged, controlled and violated by the dictatorship—and to practice art (or any cultural/intellectual practice in general) that worked in opposition to the regime meant the risk of arbitrary arrest, and of further threats such as torture and assassination. After the promulgation of AI-5, a 1968 institutional act that worsened suppression and torture practices, many artists were forced into exile, either due to the toxicity of the environment or direct threats of imprisonment.

Clark's fleeing of the dictatorship and her subsequent move to Paris in 1968 mark another moment of her working with the 'body'. At first, there is a clear 'collectivist' necessity characterising the work, which opens up micropolitical grounds more clearly, in order to pave the way to the final pieces called 'Structuring of the Self', where a vibrating, immanent body is most in evidence. From 1972 to 1976, Clark taught a course called 'The body and the space' at the Faculté d'Arts Plastiques St. Charles in the (post-1968) Sorbonne. The pieces she developed during this period were characteristically focused on collective interaction and envisaged the generation of a collective bodily experience and consciousness/perception, breaking with the subject-object dichotomy and playing out over the surface of the body. She developed a series of propositions with her group of students named *O Corpo é a Casa* (the body is the house)

(1968–1970); *Fantasmática do Corpo* (Phantasmatic of the Body), and 'Collective-Body', the latter beginning with the well-known piece 'Anthropophagic Slobber' (1973). In this piece, a group of around 60 people receive thread reels to insert on their mouths and subsequently unravel the threads over other people's bodies who remain blindfolded at the centre of the group. Wet with saliva, the massive tangle of thread is untangled before the members of the group, who share their experience verbally. Their bodies, together, open the way to the word.

The way I invite you to see this is that instead of the Other as the source of language, as we learn in psychoanalytic texts, words emerge in this collective effort, as a *co-poiesis*. Whilst this (co-poiesis) is not Clark's own phrasing, I find it alive in her creativity, and borrow from the feminist psychoanalyst Bracha Ettinger (2005, 2006, 2019), who explains it so precisely, linking it to her life's work:

> the aesthetical and ethical creative potentiality of borderlinking and of metramorphic weaving. The psychic cross-imprinting of events and the exchange of traces of mutually (but not symmetrically) subjectivizing agencies, occurring via/in a shared psychic borderspace where two or several becoming-subjectivities meet and borderlink by strings and through weaving of threads, and create singular trans-subjective webs of copoiesis composed of and by transformations along psychic strings stretched between the two or several participants of each encounter-event. Thus, a matrixial borderspace is a mutating copoietic net where co-creativity might occur. (Ettinger, 2005, p. 705)

It is in such *co-poiesis* that Clark's practice is rather unique. Her propositions challenged the problematic constitution of subjectivity via the body, collectively. Her early 1970s work sees bodies that affect other bodies in a complicated way that allow for a 'cast' to be formed on the affected body that is then 'anthropophagically' incorporated, generating a new 'becoming' (Rolnik, 2000). This trope is also particular, as Anthropophagy was an early twentieth century movement in Brazilian modernist art, of great importance. The 1922 publication of the manifesto by Oswald de Andrade in the Brazilian Modern Art Week has a strong connotation of early decolonial artistic expression. The 1922 Modern Art Week happened one hundred years after Brazil's 'independence' from Portugal. In this way, when Clark incorporates, anthropophagically, a body in her proposition, a transformation beyond a colonial Plane is implicit.

In a letter to Helio Oiticica dated 6th July 1974, Clark writes that "it is the *phantasmatics* of the body that interest me, not the body in itself" (Clark, 1974, p. 223). With regards to the process of 'Anthropophagic Slobber' she concludes: "Afterwards I ask for the *vécu* [the 'lived', in French in the original letter], which is the most important, and like this I will go on elaborating myself through the elaboration of the other..." (Clark, 1974, p. 223). This slobber seems to open up space for an ethics of a multitude of affecting 'others' that does not need to cross any anchoring transcendental referential, or Other, to be realised.

The presence of the body in this period comprises an invitation for the subject to speak *of* their body (sensations) and *through* their body, in this way, bodily experiences must give way to speech (Rivera, 2013). The parallels between this period of her work and psychoanalysis are, of course, rather potent. Indeed, during this time Lygia Clark was in analysis with Pierre Fédida in Paris, and this experiment with the '*phantasmatics* of the body' brings together the therapeutic process she is going through, a 'sewing in of the body' and an exploration of fantasies that can also be seen in her published letters exchanged with Oiticica. In the letter from the 6th of November of 1974, Lygia Clark writes extensively about fantasies that may verge on some kind of 'conscientious delirium', that are very surreal about nature, sexes, bodies, serpents coming out of her vagina, a '*tête d'abeille*' (bee head), etc., that she explored in her analysis. She writes: "In all the points of my analysis my work fits in a total manner, this is what impresses me a lot" (Clark, 1974, p. 248). The relation to the processes she has been proposing to her students and her journey in analysis with Fédida is spelled out in this long letter, where Clark is very focused on the potency of such '*phantasmatics*' of the body, as she calls it. She writes to Oiticica:

> I think that all of us who create are this and the difference between us and the psychotics is that we are capable of extending this bridge to the world by communication, or else ... ai de nós! [Untranslatable]. Through this you see that my work is my own *phantasmatic* that I give to the other, pro-

> posing that they clean it and enrich it with their own *phantasmatics*: then it is anthropophagic slobber that I vomit, that is swallowed by them and added to their own *phantasmatics* vomited once again, added until the last consequences. This is what I call a live culture and not a dead culture, which is the expression of the old support. And society, that is afraid of what is alive because it is necrophagic, it swallows everything today because everything expressed in the old support is irremediably dead. (Clark, 1974, p. 249)

It is not completely clear, certainly not fitting to any pre-established psychoanalytic concept, what Clark means by 'phantasmatics'. What we can grasp from this passage is that it relates to sensation, to exchange and possibility, to collective 'becomings'. In this same letter, Clark writes, fittingly, right after speaking of *jouissance* (in French, in an obvious reference to Lacanian psychoanalysis), that "everything is libido, everything is sensation" (Clark, 1974, p. 248). A new moment, and the one that interests this cartography the most, unfolds in her practice soon after. We may see this as an announcement of her encounter with the limits of this communication or collective experience and verbalisation model (perhaps constituted by too much of the 'dead old support', as per her letter) and her interest in a new method of propositions.

The Paris years working in groups with her students at the Sorbonne and her intense analysis with Fédida were very potent in Clark's journey and foundational to what came next, which was her establishment in the 'frontier' between art and clinic. In the end of this same November 1974 letter to Oiticica, Clark talks about the impact some of her works have had on some participants, whose lives and 'ways' have changed dramatically. She writes: "Sometimes I unblock people in one experience and, at other times, more time is needed. I had thought before being in this psychoanalysis of becoming an analyst, but now I want to continue at the 'frontier', because this is what I am and it won't do it wanting to be less frontier [*pois é isso que sou e não adianta querer ser menos fronteira*]" (Clark, 1974, p. 254). Clark returns to Brazil in 1976 and finds in her 'frontier', her borderspace, the realm to develop '*Structuring of the Self*', her last piece, carried on until she was close to the end of her life, in 1988.

Clark's contentment with the 'frontier' is very important since it challenges any easy interpretation of her project of 'abandonment of art' as 'not artistic' as such. It is not that she moved into being a therapist—she did not train, get accreditations nor affiliations with any society or school of psychoanalysis—yet she did not remain an artist in any traditional sense of the word. She became a creative clinician, or a clinical creative.

The transformative character of aesthetics and interaction were, to Clark, the real aim of her path as an artist: her abandoning of art and self-titled 'therapeutic work' in the 'Structuring of the Self' series from 1976 to 1988 worked as the climax of her practice, challenging the clinic/art divide and parking right at the frontier, the edge. In other words, Clark chooses to abandon art by not becoming exactly a psychotherapist, but instead, exploring this threshold, this in-between, as creative and generative. This abandonment or her desertion from art practice was, conversely, her greatest artistic endeavour. This work, decades later, still leaves some open questions that are relevant to the discussion around the limits of language as a Symbolic structure and of words, sounds, noise or vibrations that cross the body in the form of symptoms or affects that are central to our journey into a creative clinic for anxiety.

*Structuring of the Self* involved one-to-one exchange sessions designed to reach one person at a time, moving beyond the collective performances she was working on in France, but still challenging the status of the individual by invoking a singularity, or an individual potency, that was connected to one's experience of the world. In other words, Clark was concerned with "the reactivation of this quality of *aesthetic experience* in the receivers of her creations" (Rolnik, 2007, para. 9). Or, as Rolnik expresses it, Clark's move to this place in the 'frontier' was concerned with promoting the *Structuring of the Self*, "that is, the capacity of letting oneself be affected by the forces of objects created by the artist and the environment in which they were experienced; but above all, as a consequence, the capacity of letting oneself be affected by the forces of the environment of one's daily life" (Rolnik, 2007, para. 9). This vocabulary of 'affect' echoes what Deleuze and Guattari (1983) take from Spinoza's monism, accepting that humans and non-humans all share the same 'substance' and equally affect and are affected by each other constantly, without the need of a transcendental mediation *à la* Hegel—a discussion we will dive into together in several pit-stops along our way (Braidotti, 2006). In *Structuring of the Self*, the potency of such aesthetic experience of transformation mimicked the clinical dynamics of psychoanalysis, offering, however, more nuance into collectivity, co-construction and the commonality of the experience—or, *co-poiesis*.

Clark would see her 'patients' in her apartment in Copacabana, in Rio, for regular one-hour sessions. She would utilise her 'Objetos Relacionais' as tools for inferring sensations on the bodies of these participants. These were makeshift and cheap objects, including plastic bags, seashells, elastic bands, mattresses, etc., which were utilised to touch, cover and generate sensations on the body. Such sensations would generate affect: together they would untangle knots; they would open the unconscious through the body. The sensations facilitated by the objects and their textures and weight would open space for words that would be exchanged between Lygia Clark and her patients. The sessions were held with a frequency of up to three regular sessions a week, and the largest amount of time was dedicated to verbalising the associations stemming from the experienced sensations (Rivera, 2008). The whole session was a *co-poiesis*, or, an in-common, collective poetical construction between Clark and the patient. The aim was that after a session, the participant would then encounter reality differently and a transformation would then take place upon such encounters, as they went out into the world: the poetics of their full-void awake, activated.

## The 'full-void' Can Vibrate

What is this vibrational 'full-void' Clark taps into in her practice, and what relations to the unconscious does this presuppose? What does it have to do with our field and efforts in psychoanalysis? Or even, is there a 'full-void' of anxiety we could try to map?

Clark defines the full-void as the in/out act of reaching out to the plural possibilities awaken by the affective 'opening of the body' (Gil, 1998), a 'rite' without a 'myth' (Rolnik, 2000). In 'Nostalgia of the Body', she writes:

> What strikes me in the "inside and outside" sculpture is that it transforms my perception of myself, of my body. It changes me. I am elastic, formless, without definite physiognomy. Its lungs are mine. It's the introjection of the cosmos. And at the same time, it's my own ego crystallized as an object in space. "Inside and outside": a living being open to all possible transformations. Its internal space is an affective space. In a dialogue with my "inside and outside" work, an active subject encounters his or her own precariousness. [...] The subject discovers the ephemeral in opposition to all types of crystallization. Space is now a kind of time ceaselessly metamorphosed through action. Subject and object become essentially identified within the act. Fullness. I am overflowing with meaning. Each time I breathe, the rhythm is natural, fluid. It adheres to action. I have become aware of my "cosmic lungs." I penetrate the world's total rhythm. The world is my lung. Is this fusion death? Why does this fullness have the taste of death? I am so incredibly alive ... How to connect these two poles always? Often in my life I have discovered the identity of life and death. A discovery which nonetheless has a new flavour each time. One night, I had the perception that the absolute was this "full-void," this totality of the interior with the exterior I've spoken of so often. The "full-void" contains all potentialities. It's the act which gives it meaning. (Clark, 1994, p. 104)

We may begin by considering this collective, affective unconscious that vibrates to be a 'reverse' of psychoanalysis; a model where the body is privileged over words to the point that words barely make a difference, or even, less generously, a materialist mysticism. Yet there are clear resonances with ideas within Lacanian psychoanalysis that have been in high circulation over the past few years. Any versed Lacanian could bring out the notion of the 'speaking body', which is Jacques-Alain Miller's (2014) extrapolation of Lacan's '*parlêtre*' (speaking being) into a body that speaks as marking the twentieth-first century unconscious. Yet, the difference here is that Clark's in-out dichotomy is not resolved in a version of the subject that is 'transindividual'—which is Lacanese for being crossed by a common Symbolic that we all share and thus the subject is formed by being precisely anchored in language. Clark's 'in and out'—subject and world, flesh and unconscious—is really rather material, physical and tangible. The unconscious is bare, and accessed by sensations, not an island or a repository. The unconscious is collective, in co-production; the unconscious is affected.

Clinicians of many walks might think of Clark's technique as being just part of an artistic endeavour and not a guide for therapeutic practice. I agree and perhaps we could even assume Clark would agree too, considering she did not become an analyst herself. Yet, her work illustrates a problem in the anchoring concept of the body of the drive and the function of language in analysis as relying on foundational myths that, in one way or another, naturalise binary sexual difference and patriarchy. It is well known that Lacan's later texts were precisely veering in the direction of the limits of language, specifically through the abandonment of the Oedipal metaphor and the 'Law of the Father' as the single most important mark of subjectivation that guarantees our life 'in culture'. In psychoanalysis, such phallic Law acts as a regulator of the excess of enjoyment of the body, so a mediator of the drive and the effect of the word on the body—as such, this patriarchal universalist matrix is justified as a necessity in psychoanalysis over and over again as the guarantee 'against psychosis' (a contentious and unimaginative rulebook). In the 1970s, Lacan was leaving structuralism and its tenets and making use of topology in order to escape the limits of language in his teachings. Limits which clinical practice pushed through all the way to the fore. Until the enigmatic later teachings of Lacan in which a Real that has 'nothing to do' with the Symbolic appears, subjects are necessarily bound to the signifier and thus the 'Name-of-the-Father'. What are we left with, in our clinical practice and in theory, to think about anxiety, this point of subjective rupture, this encounter with the Real, beyond an Oedipal-Plane?

The matter of the Real of the body, as this excess in being that becomes abundant in certain symptomatic repetitions and also invoked in ideological forms of enjoyment can be encountered in several clinical and philosophical debates. To me, most attempts to grasp the 'speaking body' via this enigmatic Real that stains flesh are unsatisfactory, clinically and politically. Even bold attempts by (more) feminist (inclined) philosophers—such as what we find in Alenka Zupančič's work on sex (2017)—privilege binary sexual difference, mediated by the phallus, as the 'generative' gap of negativity in subjects (from all genders and sexes, for that matter) that leaves 'desire', or what moves us, as a negativity. My problem with that, as I will elaborate further in this book, is that we are still working within a Hegelian dialectics and therefore the possibilities for (an ecological and feminist thought of) 'becoming' are rather limited—we are stuck in a relation to a transcendental Other and a circular lack, unable to think of creative emancipation and remaining at the level of critique, as Braidotti (2013) puts it and insists on across her life's work. In Lygia Clark's terms it is rather simple: We are still stuck to the Plane.

The Hegelian dialectics inherited by Lacan assumes a division between the 'Subject' and historical time, or, assuming a Symbolic system that is mediated by the phallic law, that only re-produces subjugated subjectivities, without a chance to create something new or be in touch with any rupturing chaos outside this 'phallogocentric' system. Poststructuralist feminists such as Elizabeth Grosz and Rosi Braidotti, for example, and Suely Rolni too, reject this 'phallogocentric' subjection of subjectivity assumed as necessary mediator of desire and universalising the colonial, capitalist and patriarchal order. They propose, across decades of theoretical praxis, instead, ethical possibilities for subject formation that go beyond this beaten track. So, echoing the 1977 essay by Italian feminist Carla Lonzi (2013): 'let's spit on Hegel'—maybe with Lygia Clark's 'Anthropophagic Slobber'.

What I am trying to flesh out, with Clark's works of art as our philosophical 'relational objects', are possibilities to think of the speaking and vibrating body—the one that walks in to our clinics complaining of anxiety—outside of this Hegelian negativity and invoking a differential affirmative excess but still within psychoanalytic terms. By which I mean, still keeping psychoanalysis as primarily a practice that is radical in the context of the psy-field and mental health care but opening up to an ethical—epistemological and ontological—revision beyond the 'Plane'.

Rosi Braidotti, in her much debated book, *Transpositions*, argues for a move beyond the humanist-scented 'unitary' notion of subjectivities, and not only to a poststructuralist account at the level of Lacanian psychoanalysis—which, as she sees, still relies on 'universal values' such as the master signifier, the phallus, the Law, lack, etc.—proposing a form of 'nomadic subjectivity' instead. She is, here and across her work, inspired by ecological, feminist, post-human and post/decolonial theories that speak to Deleuze and Guattari's philosophical approach. In *Transpositions*, she spells out the necessity for taking Life as a subject, moving beyond identification and post-Hegelian dialectical models of subjectivity and negativity and towards an ethics of multiplicity and affirmation, an ethics of the 'not-one'. As she summarises:

> The focus in this line of thought is on the politics of life itself as a relentlessly generative force. The key terms in this affirmative politics are relations, endurance and radical immanence; the result is the notion of ethical sustainability. References to the non-human, inhuman or post-human play a very central role in this new ethical equation that rests on a fundamental dislocation of anthropocentric premises about agency. (Braidotti, 2010, p. 142)

Braidotti, therefore, expands accounts of a 'stranger within us' that are much indebted to psychoanalysis, and proposes an ethical encounter of affects in flux (the horizon-beyond), so not only an excess 'of me' 'in me' (or the abyss-within). She moves, like Lygia Clark, beyond the Plane. In my reading, this entails accounting not only for a Real that pertains to an excess of *jouissance* of the drive, not captured by the signifier or sublimated, that feeds symptoms, sexuality and also anxiety—as we will see in detail in Freud's early accounts of anxiety as an excess of libido. Nor is this about that Real Žižek (2010) (and his mostly male followers) so energetically defends as an inherent impossibility within the Symbolic, fitting thus within a Hegelian dialectics that situates the subject in this gap of negativity. Rather, it is about a Real that vibrates such generative encounters of the forms of Life, human and non-human, and conditions for Life, material and immaterial, situating subjectivity as a constant makeshift knotting of what extends beyond oneself. This is what Braidotti (2011, 2019) calls for in an ethics of interdependence that sits beyond identification.

Interdependence is a theme that has gained much traction among feminist scholars recently, including Silvia Federici (2019), Judith Butler (2020) and Lynne Segal (2020), to name just a few, crossing discussions that go from the climate emergency, political mobilisation and politics of care. Is there room for interdependent ethics, for multiplicity, in psychoanalysis? Or are stuck to classic Oedipal readings that will frame anxious ruptures within this particular, and problematic, view of the world?

This is where I find so much value in holding on to Lygia Clark's methods of *co-poiesis*, explicit across her later works as we have seen in this preliminary contour of our journey. It is in this nuanced and creative contribution of her practice, where multiplicity and a construction of something new realised in togetherness are proposed, that I open our suitcase. Here we are already veering away from a classic psychoanalytic method of interpreting materials brought into a session under a structured frame of references that lock all possibilities within it. Can we think, therefore, with this in mind, of an ethics of togetherness based not on the mirage of the subject but on the flux of encounters and affects? And can we think of such ethics within psychoanalysis? And more, does this inform our understanding of anxiety as an affect of rupture and eruption of the Real? Let's stay with this trouble.

## References


Braidotti, R. (2006). *Transpositions: On Nomadic Ethics*. Polity Press.

Braidotti, R. (2010). Powers of Affirmation: Response to Lisa Baraitser, Patrick Hanafin and Clare Hemmings by Rosi Braidotti. *Subjectivity, 3*, 140–148.

Braidotti, R. (2011). *Nomadic Theory. The Portable Rosi Braidotti*. Columbia University Press.

Braidotti, R. (2013, June 19). Conversation with Rosi Braidotti. *nY* [Online]. https://www.ny-web.be/artikels/conversation-rosi-braidotti/

Braidotti, R. (2019). *Posthuman Knowledge*. Polity.

Butler, J. (2020). *The Force of Nonviolence*. Verso.

Clark, L. (1974). *Cartas Lygia Clark – Hélio Oiticica 1964–1974*. ed. (1996). Editora da UFRJ.

Clark, L. (1994). Nostalgia of the Body. *October, 69*(Summer), 85–109.

Deleuze, G. M., & Guattari, F. (1983). *Anti-Oedipus – Capitalism and Schizophrenia*. University of Minnesota Press.

Ettinger, B. (2005). Copoiesis. *Ephemera, 5*(X), 703–715.

Ettinger, B. (2006). *The Matrixial Borderspace*. University of Minnesota Press.

Ettinger, B. (2019). Beyond the Death-Drive, Beyond the Life-Drive: Being-toward-Birthing with Being-toward-Birth; Copoiesis and the Matrixial Eros—Metafeminist Notes. In P. De Assis & P. Giudici (Eds.), *Aberrant Nuptials: Deleuze and Artistic Research*. Leuven University Press.
Federici, S. (2019). *Re-enchanting the World: Feminism and the Politics of the Commons*. PM Press/Kairos.
Gil, J. (1998). *Metamorphoses of the Body*. University of Minnesota Press.
Lacan, J. (1966). *Écrits*. Les Éditions du Seuil.
Lonzi, C. (2013). *Sputiamo su Hegel e altri scriti*. et al.
Miller, J. A. (2014). The Unconscious and the Speaking Body. *World Association of Psychoanalysis* [Online]. https://wapol.org/en/articulos/Template.asp?intTipoPagina=4&intPublicacion=13&intEdicion=9&intIdiomaPublicacion=2&intArticulo=2742&intIdiomaArticulo=2
Rivera, T. (2008). Ensaio sobre o espaço e o sujeito: Lygia Clark e a psicanálise. *Ágora (Rio J.), 11*(2), 219–238.
Rivera, T. (2013). *O avesso do imaginário – arte contemporânea e psicanálise*. Cosac Naif.
Rolnik, S. (2000, April 30). O corpo vibrátil de Lygia Clark. *Folha de Sao Paulo* [Online]. https://www1.folha.uol.com.br/fsp/mais/fs3004200006.htm
Rolnik, S. (2007). The Body's Contagious Memory – Lygia Clark's Return to the Museum. *Transversal* [Online]. http://eipcp.net/transversal/0507/rolnik/en
Rolnik, S. (2013a). Archive for a Work-Event: Activating the Body's Memory of Lygia Clark's Poetics and Its Context / Part 1. *Manifesta* #13 [Online]. http://www.manifestajournal.org/issues/fungus-contemporary
Rolnik S. (2013b). Archive for a Work-Event, Activating the Body's Memory of Lygia Clark's Poetics and Its Context, Part II. *Manifesta* #14 [Online]. http://www.manifestajournal.org/issues/souvenirs-souvenirs
Segal, L., Chatzidakis, A., Hakim, J., Littler, J., & Rottenberg, C. (2020). *The Care Manifesto*. Verso.
Žižek, S. (2010). *Interrogating the Real*. Continuum.
Zupančič, A. (2017). *What Is Sex?* MIT Press.

# 3

# The Production of Anxiety

During the first months of the Covid-19 pandemic, prescriptions for antidepressant, anti-anxiety and anti-insomnia drugs were reported to have risen by 21% in the United States.[1] In the United Kingdom, early reports also suggested demand increased between 10 and 15% for antidepressant drugs in pharmacies in the first months of the crisis (Sharma, 2020). The Office of National Statistics (ONS) reported that half of the British population experienced 'high anxiety' during the weeks of Spring 2020 lockdown (ONS, 2020).

Whilst uncertainty, vulnerability and stress, coupled with precarity, lace the impoverishment of overall wellbeing in critical times, what would be the line dividing a pathological disorder and a healthy, if anything, reaction to torment in light of troubling circumstances? In order to gauge the status and politics of the contemporary pathologising (and individualising and de-politicising) of anxious distress and the possibilities of our relation with it, we must begin by asking other elementary questions. If anxiety is negative, then how much anxiety is too much? And how could

[1] According to the Report 'America's State of Mind', published in April 2020 by the private healthcare provider Express Scripts, anti-anxiety benzodiazepines prescription rose 34% during the first month of Covid-19 crisis, whilst antidepressant SSRI/SNRI pills saw an increase in 18% of prescriptions filed by health care providers across the USA. Retrieved from https://www.express-scripts.com/corporate/americas-state-of-mind-report?mod=article_inline.



A. C. Minozzo, *Anxiety as Vibration*, Studies in the Psychosocial,
https://doi.org/10.1007/978-3-031-62856-6_3

we measure it? The classification of psychological suffering stumbles upon the challenge of quantifying the 'un-quantifiable' through the systematic categorising and description of affective and mental states and their transformation into illnesses and disorders.

In this chapter, we will think about anxiety through a critical recent history of its diagnosis and treatment in the context of psychological care. This will help us to gauge the dimension of our anxious troubles a little better. By unpacking the strategies employed by mainstream psychiatry in the Diagnostic and Statistical Manual of Mental Disorders (DSM), published by the American Psychiatric Association (APA) since the mid-twentieth century, it is possible to unveil the dynamics of a reduction of the subject to a productive-biomedicalised body in the last decades. Such a process echoes a mode of governance that finds its realisation not only in the clinic but also in contemporary modes of consumption and discourses and policies of wellbeing. What becomes apparent is a process of quantification, qualification and management of affects; or, as I propose here, an affective-politics that assembles body and psyche in a particular mode of alienation—an 'estrangement'.

This diagnostic culture, inaugurated in the late-1970s, is framed by a logic of categorisation and control of the body, which becomes a particularly complex locus of 'dividualisation' (Deleuze, 1992)—a concept Gilles Deleuze utilised to address the mode of subjective production of the contemporary society of control, entailing a loss of the possibility of experience of subjective truth in symptoms that anchor the psychoanalytic conception of anxiety. Deleuze's mapping allows us to grapple with the current efforts of management of anxiety and management of the body that culminates in what pharmaceutical lobbying calls 'a silent epidemic', with circa 20% of the US population, for example, experiencing 'pathological' or 'not-normal' levels of anxiety (Cooke, 2013; ADAA, 2021; NIHM, 2021). Such mechanisms and fantasies of taming and controlling the body through consumption, public policy or medication, relate to Michel Foucault's archaeology of 'biopower', once the study of power and the body in his work entails the investigation of the "modes of objectification which transform human beings into subjects" (Foucault, 1982, p. 777). Foucault (1982) summarises the three 'types' of objectifications in this process of subjectivation explored throughout his life's work. They are: “the modes of inquiry which try to give themselves the status of sciences” (Foucault, 1982, p. 777); ‘dividing practices’ in which the “subject is either divided inside himself or divided from others” (Foucault, 1982, p. 778); and “the way a human being turns himself into a subject” (Foucault, 1982, p. 778). Language, scientific knowledge, discourse, governmentality and subjectivation are features of our analysis of the status of anxiety, revealing a dividualising biopolitical modulation of affect—or, a systematic estrangement that anchors care, further alienating suffering from its singular and contextual roots. The landscape is grim.

## Unwanted Anxiety

The British Office for National Statistics (ONS) has been putting into practice a governmental policy-planning programme entitled ‘Measuring National Well-being’ (MNW) since November 2010. By asking a set of four questions, their aim is to “develop and publish an accepted and trusted set of National Statistics which help people understand and monitor well-being” (ONS, 2018) and by ‘wellbeing’ they understand: “‘how we are doing’ as individuals, as communities and as a nation, and how sustainable this is for the future” (ONS, 2018). The project follows the contemporary tendency that Christian Dunker, a Brazilian psychoanalyst, describes as a move guiding public policy through a ‘diagnosis’-based modus operandi (Dunker, 2015). “To diagnose,” he writes, “has become one of the activities most specifically valued in our current form of life” (Dunker, 2015, p. 20). If we look into the four questions being asked by the ‘Quality of Life Team’ to thousands of citizens in the UK in the past decade, the connection between that and a ‘diagnostic culture’ becomes clearer. They are:

“Overall, how satisfied are you with your life nowadays?”
“Overall, to what extent do you feel the things you do in your life are worthwhile?”
“Overall, how happy did you feel yesterday?”
“Overall, how anxious did you feel yesterday?” (ONS, 2018).

Whilst 'positivity' is measured in terms of happiness, satisfaction and purpose, the sole question qualifying 'negativity' of the wellbeing experience is measured by the appearance of anxiety. Feeling anxious, it seems, connotes a status of 'ill-being'.

Such a qualification of anxiety as negative and undesirable reveals crossings between the universes of inside and outside the clinic that have merged discourses, governmentality, treatment and consumption into the same 'diagnostic'-logic in which wellbeing, or feeling well, feeling good, means not feeling anxious. Dunker calls this logical/ideological expansion a '*diagnóstica*' [in Portuguese], a term he summarises as the 'diagnosis-like' frame offering the "condition of possibilities of diagnostic systems" (Dunker, 2015, p. 20) to a context that is outside the initial scope of such diagnostic logic. A '*diagnóstica*', therefore, is characterised by a system of framing, recognising and cataloguing other aspects of life that exceed clinical diagnosis and treatment but still remaining in a format informed by the same dynamics that frame the clinic, or the contemporary medico-scientific and therapeutic field of psy (Rose, 1996). In this sense, anxiety is inserted within the public cultural discourse following a process of pathologising and symptomatic isolation that is present in the psychiatric diagnostic context. As such, this logic seeps into the public sphere as a measure and indicator of an 'unwanted' status of being, as seen in the ONS wellbeing questionnaire. Anxiety is being produced by the *diagnóstica* that frames it at the same time. Under such lenses, the grammar of the Diagnostic and Statistical Manual of Mental Disorders (DSM) allows us to grapple the mechanisms of production of our relation with the affect of anxiety.

In the early to mid-twentieth century, owing to the psychoanalytic influence in psychiatry, the widespread nonspecific naming of the modern sense of discontent, or *Unbehagen*, was 'neurotic anxiety'. In this period "anxiety and its sibling condition, 'neuroses', became the central themes of what came to be called the stress tradition" (Horwitz, 2010, p. 113), thus revealing a certain trend of 'pathologising' anxiety, despite anxiety being considered a common affliction of the post-World War II world. However ubiquitous or familiar to the post-war subject, anxiety was also the main category for discriminating in the clinic what was 'normal' and what was 'pathological' in that same period. Depression, at that point, as Horwitz (2010, 2013) defends, was 'in practice'—and by that he means, in the practice of psychiatrists in the United States—more commonly associated with the psychotic sphere and was a characteristic diagnosis reserved for severe melancholic cases of hospitalised patients. This trend will come to a halt towards the later decades of the twentieth century precisely, as we will see in what follows, due to a disappearance of the influence of psychoanalytic theory in the field of mainstream psychiatry. Before the 1980s, psychiatric diagnoses "reflected the centrality of the 'psychoneuroses', which were grounded in anxiety" (Horwitz, 2010, p. 115) and the first two editions of the DSM, from 1952 and 1968 respectively, are considered to be the most flavoured by psychodynamics—the type of psychotherapeutic knowledge that takes into account the dynamic unconscious of psychoanalysis. From the third edition onwards, however, there is an increased trend in further categorising mental illness in search of a 'reliable' efficiency in diagnosis that culminates in the fifth and most recent edition of the manual, the DSM-V, from 2013, with its bulk of over nine hundred pages of 'disorders' and their respective diagnostic checklists (Vanheule, 2014; Ehrenberg, 2009; Herzberg, 2009). This change in approach will reshape the status of anxiety and, consequently, promote a biological narrative of depression in the turn of the twenty-first century. It also presents us with a paradigm shift in regards to the quantification of the body, psyche and affect, maintaining the status of 'ruptures' and suffering as ever more individualised and alienated from the one suffering and their context.

The process of mapping and categorising mental states and affects and transforming them into recognisable symptoms is at the heart of the birth of the DSM, making it into a quantifying *dispositif par excellence*, informing what Felicity Callard (2014) calls a 'mediated' relation to diagnosis. The DSM emerges as a 'promise', at least, of a more 'pragmatic' and 'detailed' approach to substitute the then existing diagnostic forms, which were mostly based on prototypical descriptions and hypothetical case-studies rather than 'checklists'. The prototypical approach was already seen in earlier key texts of psychiatry such as Philippe Pinel's *A Treatise on Insanity*, from (1806), where distinctions of 'treatable' and 'untreatable' patients and principles of moral and medical treatments of what he called insanity were laid out systematically. This was despite the fact that Pinel had "a single view of madness, characterised by many symptoms" (Ehrenberg, 2009, p. 36), rather than 'different types of madness', as we can see in a psychoanalytic and psychodynamic approach that divided, at a basic level, psychoses and neuroses as different structures. In the early twentieth century, Pinel's approach was still dominant in psychiatry, making use of clinical vignettes of patients' cases that guided doctors by some type of comparison. Psychoanalysis relied on clinical analysis and conjectural 'judgement', rather than on a clear-cut dividing line between what caused or classified a symptom as pathological or even as a symptom in the first place (Vanheule, 2014). A similar reliance on the doctor in question was present in the traditions that favoured a prototypical approach. It was in part as a promise to facilitate these individual judgements on the side of the doctor that the first major manual of mental illness was published in the United States by the APA in 1918. The 'Statistical Manual for the Use of Institutions for the Insane' was published ten different times before being substituted by the first edition of the DSM, in 1952.

At the time, however, different authors would already have diverging opinions on mental illness, and founding heavy-names of the psy-disciplines such as Emil Kraepelin and Eugen Bleuler, for example, presented contrasting views over the focus either on biological components or, rather, more 'holistic' aetiological approaches. Psychiatry was a mixed field and "in the 1950s and 1960s, while psychoanalysis occupied the commanding heights of American psychiatry" (Scull, 2019, p. 133), the first edition of the DSM was published. This first edition "reflected the movement of psychiatric practice from state mental hospitals to outpatient treatment and thus paid more attention to the psychoneuroses" (Horwitz & Wakefield, 2012, p. 93) instead of psychosis, the latter being more frequently 'reserved' to hospital wards. The paradigm of the asylum and of a medicalised culture that excluded the insane from society, as explored in depth in Foucault's (2008a) work on psychiatric power and biopolitics, starts cracking from this point onwards. Anxiety, therefore, was a common handle in clinical practice in the mid-twentieth century due to the influence of psychoanalysis and what we may call 'everyday' madness and suffering (Crocq, 2015, 2017). Anxiety, importantly, was seen not a disorder in itself, but as a signal of something else that had to be treated on a contextual and individual basis.

The influence of North American psychiatry is politically relevant because such paradigmatic frameworks have reflected on systems of classification and of quantification across the globe. In the 1950s and 1960s, the then dominant group at the American Psychiatric Association (APA), under the auspices of Adolf Meyer, conferred their psychodynamic preference on the manual, and such psychoanalytic 'flavour' was not lost even with the changes imposed by the following second version of the DSM, published in the late 1960s (Scull, 2019). The second edition was published after the release of the 6th edition of the International Classification of Diseases (ICD), published by the World Health Organization (WHO) that had been formed in 1948; this sixth edition inaugurated the ICD model existent to date. For those of you unfamiliar with all such acronyms, ICD codes are used every day across the globe in health appointments when making a diagnosis, charging health insurances, creating epidemiological maps and informing public health policy. In the 1960s, therefore, envisaging a pairing of the DSM with the ICD-6, as this was the first of its kind to list mental health disorders, the APA launched the DSM II. The 1968 edition "did not make any major changes in the account of the anxiety disorders or in the pivotal role of anxiety in psychopathology. It maintained anxiety as the key aspect of the psychoneuroses" (Horwitz & Wakefield, 2012, p. 95). Anxiety was still a central component of the frame that conferred a diagnostic platform to the then dominant diagnoses at the period, but that was about to change in the next decade.

A contrasting view to the usually widely accepted understanding of the influence of the DSM-III in the boom of psychopharmaceutic treatment, as we will see next, is offered by Metzl (2003). In his book *Prozac on the Couch*, he argues that it was the Freudian psychoanalytic culture of 'blaming' anxious suffering on poor or disturbed mothering that contributed a vocabulary to the popularisation of tranquilising pills through women's magazines in the United States in the 1950s. Arguing that "anxiety was the pressure of keeping intact the structure in which the doctor prescribes and the patient ingests" (Metzl, 2003, p. 124), Metzl localises in psychoanalysis the roots of later biological psychiatry in which the doctor prescribes the pill that cures. Whilst Metzl offers a compelling critique of the gendered language of both mass media and of psychoanalytic texts, rightly identifying the misogyny and biologism of Freudian and post-Freudian writing, little context of the psycho-politics of diagnosis is provided. Therefore, whilst carving a rather convincing argument about who gets excluded and on what grounds from ideals of normality, sanity or wellbeing, Metzl too quickly diagnoses psychoanalysis without looking, for example, to other countries where the psychoanalytic discourse might have been equally or more widespread in the early twentieth century. The author also fails to critically address the contributions of Freudian ideas about psychotherapeutic 'talking cures', where psychic life is implicated in discourse rather than reduced to a purely medicalised solution. Consequently, neither his understanding of 'Freudian biology' nor of the specificities of anxiety versus depression as paradigms of suffering is particularly clear. For as much as the hegemonic power of psychoanalytic discourses within psychiatry in the USA until the 1950s is noticeable, it can hardly account for the rise of depression in the following decades, as we will see next.

## The DSM-III and the Disappearance of Anxiety

The third edition of the DSM, published in 1980, inaugurated a decisive distancing from the psychoanalytic approach and, with that, managed to re-signify the status of anxiety. This proved to be critical in inaugurating a novel kind of quantification of affect, favouring biological explanations of psychic distress and giving birth to depression as the illness of the century (Verhaeghe, 2008). To comprehend the motor of this change from the ubiquity of anxiety towards mass-depression diagnoses there are some elements to consider of the politics of psychiatry at the time and also the influence of products being marketed by the pharmaceutical industry (Scull, 2019). Such factors had an important role in producing the 'grammar' of anxiety in the last half of the twentieth century. What we see as a drastic change implemented in the DSM-III is a moving away from the prototype-based model and an introduction of the checklist-logic of diagnosis. A group of biological psychiatrists based at Washington

University in St. Louis, United States, led by Robert Spitzer and known as neo-Kraepelinian—for their biological inclination—was tasked with the formulation of the third edition of the manual; their core interest was to define psychiatry as a medical discipline (Shorter, 2005). This alignment with the medical discourse was achieved by the introduction of a new system based on a list of criteria, "Spitzer's task force was a political animal, and its aim was to simplify the diagnostic process by reducing it to a tick-the-boxes approach" (Scull, 2019, p. 172). This system inaugurated in the third edition of the manual is still guiding its current version, the fifth, since such a checklist approach that classifies, qualifies and quantifies is seen as more 'scientific' than narrative models of treatment that preceded it. Checklists, in fact, seem to be far from going anywhere in mental health care.

In this new model, anxiety no longer features as an aspect of psychic experience and neurotic distress, rather, each 'type' of suffering is allocated into an individual category. Anxiety now is divided into subcategories of phobias, separation anxiety, panic disorder and so on (Shorter, 2005; Harrington, 2019), leaving the category of General Anxiety Disorder, or GAD, as the only nonspecific category of diagnosis. GAD could only be 'ticked' however, when no other type of anxiety was present. This move alone demarcates a significant effort in qualifying the affect of anxiety. Conversely, the broad category of Major Depressive Disorder, or MDD, appears as the go-to general diagnosis of distress (Mojtabai & Olfson, 2008). The results of this 'grammatical' shift are critical. Whilst the numbers of diagnoses of depression in the USA during the 1960s accounted for roughly one third of the diagnoses related to anxiety, in the 1980s depression overtook anxiety. This trend only intensified in the following years and according to the USA National Centre for Health Statistics, by the early-2000s the proportion of anxiety versus depression diagnoses shifted completely: from about fifty million overall yearly diagnoses of mental health a year, over twenty million were of depression whilst only six million were diagnosed as anxiety (Herzberg, 2009).

Depression travels, then, as we are able to trace historically, from belonging mostly to the melancholic and hospitalised world all the way into ordinary experience. It moves from being a peripheral category into being a dominant diagnosis of the 'stress tradition' (Crocq, 2015). Alongside the moving away from the anxiety-paradigm of the psychoneuroses that marked so heavily the psychodynamic approach of the earlier versions of the DSM, by the late 1970s 'depression' as an overarching category itself also appears to "fit the professionally desirable conception of a severe and specific disease that could be associated with biological causes" (Horwitz, 2010, p. 123). Therefore, it served well the then dominant group within the hegemonic forces of the psy-field, whilst it also brought the roots of 'discontent' close to the body, to the organism. In simple terms, the 'new malaise' favoured biologism, in contrast with a hard to measure psychoanalytic neurotic anxiety, and it also served, by consequence, the thriving pharmaceutical industry (Herzberg, 2009; Harrington, 2019).

## The Social Life of Depression

Beyond the United States and beyond the close-circuit of psychiatry comparable currents were being established. The sociologist Alain Ehrenberg writes of a similar flow across the Atlantic, in France, demonstrating analogous shifts between anxiety and depression from the mid to the end of the twentieth century. He points out that "according to the *credes* (Centre d'études et de documentation sur la santé), between the beginning of the 1980s and the beginning of the 1990s, the rate of depression increased 50 percent in France" (Ehrenberg, 2009, p. 181). What Ehrenberg offers as an interesting contextual analysis of the soaring numbers of depression diagnoses and, consequently, the changes in the meaning of anxiety as a symptom or a disorder, is the accompanying ideological shift marked by the definition of the subject of depression and its supposed ideal counterpart, the 'autonomous' and 'emancipated' subject. The rise of the autonomous individual from the late 1970s that was being slowly announced through the cultural shifts that followed the Second World War is, according to Ehrenberg, an important factor in the emergence of depression as a representation of a depleted individual that finds itself powerless, facing a demand of 'autonomy' and 'emancipation' that was accompanied by a contrasting sense of 'freedom'—however illusory and constricted this 'freedom' to be oneself was and still is. In this context, anxiety appears only as a consequence of this overall sense of 'unfitness'. It appears as an anxiety signalling the possibility of failure to truly correspond to such demands (Ehrenberg, 2009), yet, peripheral if compared to depression.

The changes in (some parts of Western) society that followed the 1960s—e.g. countercultural movements, civil rights movements, recognition movements, etc.—in various forms in different territories and contexts are, for Ehrenberg, a driving power behind a new, as he puts it, "strange obsession with being entirely oneself" (Ehrenberg, 2009, p. 135). Depression, as a polar opposite of such aspirational emancipation, appeared as a convenient representation "to describe the problems raised by this new normality" (Ehrenberg, 2009, p. 135), the 'normality' being therefore 'emancipation'. For, as he points out, "individual sovereignty was not only a relaxation of external constraints; everyone could also take the concrete measure of the inner burden it brought into being" (Ehrenberg, 2009, p. 135). If Freudian psychoanalysis marked the late nineteenth century and early twentieth century neurotic subject, characterised by repression and guilt in its Victorian and bourgeois Viennese universe, the late twentieth century saw a different problem emerging, and that was, for Ehrenberg, the omnipotence that shadowed emancipation.

> After the Second World War, depression separates itself from melancholia. Depression travels between two versions of the difficult task of being well: (1) anxiety, which indicated that I am crossing into forbidden territory and am becoming divided, a pathology of guilt, an illness of conflict; and (2) exhaustion, which tired me out, empties me, and makes me incapable of action—a pathology of responsibility, an illness of inadequacy.
>
> These two versions of wellness accompany the emergence of a new era of the self, who is no longer either the complete individual of the eighteenth century; or the split individual of the end of the nineteenth century; rather, she is the emancipated individual. Becoming ourselves made us nervous, being ourselves makes us depressed. The anxiety of being oneself hides behind the weariness of the self. (Ehrenberg, 2009, pp. 43–44)

Brazilian psychoanalyst Maria Rita Kehl has a complementary insight into the matter of the rise of depression in the twentieth century and in her book *O Tempo e o Cão* (or 'Time and the Dog', in English), she depicts the depressed subject as occupying the place of the melancholic in previous centuries. Depression is, according to Kehl, a 'positioning'—or an 'unconscious choice', in the psychoanalytic sense—of the subject in face of an 'impossible' Other, representing a 'social symptom'. She argues that "the potential of analysis of the social bond represented since antiquity by melancholies has nowadays been relocated to the field of depressions" (Kehl, 2015, p. 49). The contrast between melancholia and depression taken up by Kehl follows a Lacanian reading of Freud's work on melancholia, that situates it, as she explains in the book, 'more to the side' of psychosis (Kehl, 2015) than neurosis, as Freud had initially marked melancholia—and psychosis—as 'narcissistic neuroses'. In this manner, to Kehl, in simple terms, the melancholic 'in its time' was subjected to a fundamental loss marked in the relation with a 'mOther' that was not desiring, not castrated, thus, not offering a 'place' for this subject. Subjectivity and the Other in a period that we could perhaps succinctly call 'modern' were crossed by the discontent of melancholia, of the loss of this possibility of having a place in the world, according to Kehl—a view shared in a way by other feminists, nonetheless (Sprengnether, 1995). The depressed, in her view, is claiming a 'place' in light of a different Other in our times. Furthering such acknowledgement of a sort of 'social life of depression', Kehl observes that "the rise in the incidence of the so-called 'depressive disorders', since the last three decades of the twentieth century, indicates that we should try to question what do the depressions have to say to us, from the place that was previously occupied by the old manifestations of melancholy, as symptoms of the contemporary forms of '*mal-estar*' [the Portuguese translation of Freud's *Unbehagen*]" (Kehl, 2015, p. 49). Indeed, statistical patterns of diagnosis are revealing of shifts in society; however, the production of the diagnostic categories must be considered carefully as actively productive of such shifts. This means that studies considering the rise in certain patterns of diagnosis need to also acknowledge the fact that the politics of generating the manuals, categories and checklists utilised in diagnoses will be reflected in the collective experience such studies are analysing. For instance: peaks in diagnoses of depression can offer clues to the interpretation that society is 'more depressed'; however, this straightforward analysis is superficial if it does not take into account the factors informing these mass diagnoses. In this sense, Kehl's book bypasses the equally statistical and data-rich analysis observed by Horwitz (2010), for instance, that the rise in 'depression' followed from a previous mass pathologising of anxiety and pointing out that all that anxiety, therefore, cannot have suddenly just 'vanished'.

Kehl brings in anxiety only as a part of depression, openly limiting her attempts at elaborating on the impact of psychiatric diagnosis or even the pharmaceutic industry over the rise in the numbers of 'depressed people' across the globe. Diverging slightly from Ehrenberg, whilst quoting similar patterns of diagnosis in Brazil[2] to those of France and the USA, Kehl's 'negative' of the depressive subject is the capitalist 'productive subject'. Depression, depletion and under—or no—productivity are the markers of what is unacceptable or at least undesirable to the maintaining of the capitalist system in its neoliberal turn (Sadowsky, 2021). In this light, a state of 'excess', the opposite of 'depletion', could be interpreted as more favourable to this neoliberal project. However, by looking through anxiety carefully in the psychoanalytic writings of Freud and Lacan, a paradoxical state of excess [of tension], that may prompt one to act at the same time as generating a total lack of action, in stillness, is found as pertaining to the sphere of anxiety. An anxious subject is not necessarily productive, nor necessarily unproductive. We may perhaps say that the anxious subject is a subject that does not 'fit' into a particular capitalist project perfectly, yet, it does not 'not fit' either. To explore these paradoxical remarks, it is useful to comprehend not only what it 'means' to be categorised or diagnosed as depressed or anxious, rather, we must not separate this questioning from enquiring into 'how' these categories are formulated and what revolves around such 'grammar'.

---

[2] Kehl describes the patterns of diagnosis of depression in Brazil as follows: "In Brazil, circa 17 million people were diagnosed as depressive in the first years of the twenty-first century. According to a reportage of the newspaper Valor Economico, in regards to the twentieth anniversary of Prozac, the market of antidepressants has been growing in the country by 22% each year, what represents an annual gross movement of 320 million dollars" (Kehl, 2015, p. 50).

Kehl's approach via the 'undesirable' subject for neoliberal capitalism has important theoretical resonances and interesting clinical value. As she explains in this piece, in the clinic, encountering depressed subjects has become increasingly more frequent and it is by offering them a different set up to negotiate their relation to this initially 'impossible' Other, as well as to re-inscribe their *jouissance* in this relation of desire and demand that analysis can offer something potent in the face of depression. However, this focus on the 'depressed' subject, as if this category has some 'objective bearings' on reality, leaves the debate around anxiety aside or at least in a peripheral space as if it 'suddenly' vanished from collective experience upon the rise of the diagnosis of depression. It is crucial, thus, when still engaging with the reverberations of capitalism and social arrangements in the clinic, to understand the project of privatisation of suffering and its naming, framing, categorisation and qualification up close, mapping its relation to profit and private and public institutions, as well as the ideological echoes of such *diagnóstica*. In other words, it is crucial to consider the grammar for such inscriptions and recognition of suffering.

## Quantifying Affect: From Discontent to Medication

As early as the 1950s and 1960s, experimentations with psychopharmacological drugs and the modulation of anxiety can be observed. Felicity Callard (2016) offers a comprehensive study of the relation between agoraphobia and the still popular category 'panic disorder' in the collaboration between the North-American psychiatrists Donald Klein and Max Fink. Klein was part of the DSM-III taskforce, where anxiety is, for the first time, dissolved into different categories. His particular contribution was that his work on medicalising and defining what 'panic' looked like, in contrast with agoraphobia and a more 'general' anxiety, informed the alliance between segmentation of symptoms, drug effects and a new status for anxiety. Callard (2016) recounts Klein and Fink's treatment of patients between the years of 1958–1959 with Imipramine—'the first tricyclic antidepressant' (Callard, 2016, p. 214); such experiments led Klein to argue "that drug action allowed the observation of two ontologically distinct kinds of anxiety (anticipatory anxiety and panic) that had been conflated in earlier models and theorisations of anxiety" (Callard, 2016, p. 204). Psychopharmaceutic thinking, or this artificial pharmacological paradigm, was thus introduced as an anchor to a biological psychiatric definition of symptoms, disorders and, overall, affect and anxiety.

The 'fall' of anxiety thus hardly represents the diminishing of anxious states in the experience of individuals, rather, it is a 'fall' reliant not solely on diluted socio-political changes and their production of subjectivity, but also on the politics of the systems of diagnosis and treatments and their representation of contemporary capitalist interests. The publication of the DSM-III and the shift towards a biological cause of distress facilitate a 'chemical imbalance' narrative that was accompanied by mass marketing campaigns aimed at both the general public and clinicians as well as profitable drug patents (Shorter, 2009; Whitaker, 2010). The most famous case study of the sort is the 1987 pill launched by Eli Lilly: Prozac. Within ten years of its launch, 10% of the North American population was already taking it (Segal, 2017). In the USA, in 1988, the National Institute of Mental Health (NIMH) launched the 'Depression Awareness, Recognition, and Treatment Program' (DART), and Prozac (fluoxetine) featured in 8 million brochures and 200,000 posters sponsored by its manufacturer (Segal, 2017). The serotogenic rebalance becomes the pharmacological promise of the following decades, giving Prozac many successful companion drugs known as Selective Serotonin Reuptake Inhibitors (SSRIs), such as citalopram, escitalopram, sertraline or paroxetine. Highly promoted through marketing, these drugs are still dominant in prescription not only for MDD as well as 'anxieties' and even GAD. Well known for not causing side-effects and addiction as harsh as those caused by earlier tranquilisers and anxiolytics such as Miltown (meprobamate), Valium and Librium (benzodiazepines), popular during the 1950s and 1960s, SSRIs benefit from a marketed reputation of being 'effective' and even 'harmless'. It is only more recently and slowly, that the dangers of withdrawal and of severe side-effects of SSRI and SNRI antidepressants have been researched, impacting public health recommendations of disclosure of withdrawal harm upon prescription in general medical practice. In 2019 the British Royal College of Psychiatrists (2019) officially took a critical position in relation to withdrawal of anti-depressants in their recommendations to NICE—the National Institute for Health and Care Excellence.

What is curious is that anxiety returns 'blurred' within depression through psycho-pharmaceutical treatments named 'anti-depressant' (Herzberg, 2009). Such is the terminology factor in the fall and rise of certain diagnosis that in an article in *The Guardian*, from June 2017, the then dean of The Royal College of Psychiatrists, Dr Kate Lovett, is quoted affirming that: "Antidepressants are used in the treatment of both depression and anxiety disorders. They are an evidence-based treatment for moderate to severe depression and their prescription should be reviewed regularly in line with clear national guidance" (Campbell, 2017). Under such discourse, as stressed in the 'scientific' tone of an adjective such as 'evidence based', contemporary antidepressants work in a 'versatile' fashion, both when you are 'up' or 'down', anxious or depressed. The first patented drug to benefit from this shift back to a 'new age of anxiety diagnosis', in which anxiety returns in a biologised form, was Paxil (paroxetine), approved in the United States in 1999 for the treatment of Social Anxiety Disorder, known as SAD, and in 2001 for General Anxiety Disorder (Rose, 2006). The product, only a decade later, generated three billion dollars in sales a year (Horwitz, 2010) and a good part of such 'success', especially in the USA, is due to the heavy television advertising of the drug promoted by GlaxoSmithKline (and its pre-merger name SmithKline Beecham) "suggesting to individuals that their worry and anxiety at home and at work might not be because they are just worriers but because they are suffering from a treatable condition. 'Paxil … Your life is waiting'" (Rose, 2007, p. 213) read the adverts.

When the then SmithKline Beecham pharmaceutic company was seeking FDA (USA Food and Drug Administration) licensing for Paxil, social anxiety disorder was still not as widely known by the general public and to tackle this 'problem', the company "launched a public advertising campaign called 'Imagine Being Allergic to People.' The campaign included the 'cobbling together' of a patient advocacy group called the Social Anxiety Disorder Coalition" (Harrington, 2019, p. 568). A similar PR strategy to promote the 'chemical imbalance' narrative of mental distress was employed by Pfizer in 1999, when marketing the SSRI Zoloft for PTSD, Post-Traumatic Stress Disorder, for which they hired the public relations firm Chandler Chicco Agency to form the advocacy group 'PTSD Alliance' (Harrington, 2019). Other drugs have been approved for the treatment of anxiety in its many categories as stated in the most recent editions of the DSM since the late 1990s. Zoloft (sertraline) and Effexor (venlafaxine, officially a serotonin and norepinephrine reuptake inhibitor, or SNRI) have also been marketed for PTSD and GAD respectively. The DSM-III and following IV and V breakdown of anxiety into different disorders amplified the market scope for Big Pharma, accordingly, "the strategy of repurposing old drugs for new disorders (that, in many cases, people had not known they had) was highly successful. U.S. sales of SSRIs picked up again dramatically, peaking in 2008 with revenues of $12 billion" (Harrington, 2019, p. 571).

The profitability behind the shift towards a checklist-approach of diagnosis also reveals a tragic unethical mingling of Big Pharma and governing bodies. For the latest edition of the DSM, for example, the DSM-V, "it was reported that the pharmaceutical industry was responsible for half of the APA's $50 million budget, and that eight of the eleven-strong committee which advised on diagnostic criteria had links to pharmaceutical firms" (Davies, 2015, p. 124). The ethically problematic conflict of interests present in the structure that creates diagnostic criteria, funds research and, in general terms, produces the 'grammar of suffering', reveals "the entanglement of psychic maximization and profit maximization" (Davies, 2015, p. 124), crossing through the vocabulary available for identifying and recognising mental suffering.

There are other links between this model of diagnosis and the operative global financial capitalist system, once a manual such as the DSM comes to operate as a neo-colonising discourse through the imposition of its frameworks of categorisation of psychic experience (Sadowsky, 2021). This relation is clearer if we look into the DSM's presence around the world. Despite being a North American psychiatric manual, the DSM has its scope and influence more 'globally'. If at the start of the DSM project and with the DSM-II in particular, there was a preoccupation in matching the 'international' standards of the ICD, after the third edition of the DSM, the 'power' shifts hands. With the publication of the

DSM-III, in 1980 things move to the opposite direction and the ICD goes on to follow the trends in diagnosis already present in the DSM. Until the ICD-9, from 1975, the umbrella-terms of 'psychosis' and 'neurosis' were present. During this period, in the United States, an extraordinary issue of the international manual called ICD-9-CM (with CM standing for 'clinical modifications') was launched, opening path for the upcoming hybridity in codes. In the following version of the international manual, the first post-DSM-III, the ICD-10, from 1992, a longer list of very specific and detailed types of 'disorders' appears, reflecting the categories' checklist system (Shorter, 2009). Despite the gaps in publishing time, both manuals present a similar development of the trends in diagnosis, especially in terms of moving away from a psychodynamic-influenced language and a shift towards further divisions and categories. Ingrid Palmary and Brendon Barnes (2015) comment on the 'hegemonic' power of the North American psychiatric manual in their study of critical psychology and diagnoses in African countries. Reproducing colonial dynamics, as seen in Nigeria for example, the DSM "was consistently used in such a way that the clinician could devalue the meanings given by the client and focus only on those parts of the narrative that were congruent with the way mental health was understood in the DSM" (Palmary & Barnes, 2015, p. 398). They add: "In this way, Western psychological knowledge is reproduced as the true focus whilst local knowledge is rendered irrelevant or at most a cultural variation" (Palmary & Barnes, 2015, p. 398).

This 'imported' and 'exported' grammar of suffering that is at the core of the project of the ICD for public health, whilst crossed by the logic of the DSM, also represents a colonising 'globalisation' of the manners of suffering that accompanied the globalisation of financial capital within the neoliberal ideology. It is worth mentioning that along the terminology of 'global health' and several private-public and philanthropic capitalist efforts, the USA is still the largest donor to the WHO yearly budgets. The subject 'of' neoliberal capitalism becomes, through such diagnostic systems and multinational pharmaceutical corporations, a 'global' paradigm, and the potentiality of affects such as anxiety or the possibilities involved in experiencing psychic distress are erased systematically by the hegemonic practices in the field of psy, serving the 'powers' of 'globalised' financialisation of human capital. Affect is divided and conquered in a neo-colonising effort.

The connection of this diagnostic culture to neoliberalism goes further and deeper, as we are taken to an affective-politics that produces a biologised negativity in anxiety and profits from it (Guéry & Deleule, 2014). In this manner, when we accept that the DSM provides categories for recognition of distress, "it must be recognised that this language is not neutral and value-free but rather reflects a dominant ideological rhetoric of the specific epoch, in this case the crisis in welfarism and the emergence of neoliberalism" (Cohen, 2016, p. 79). Neoliberalism and a broader culture organised by the criteria of performance/production see a reverberation in the field of psy through the relationship established with medication. What are these pills for? "Cure, palliative treatment or doping?" (Dunker, 2015, p. 23). To put it simply: where do we draw the line between the use of a substance to ease a painful difficulty/suffering and eliminate 'all' suffering and discomfort? Or even, when does medication become what doping is to an athlete, an aid to up one's performances and increase benefits? Therefore, a 'diagnostic grammar'—informed and formed by the 'alliances' between hegemonic powers in the field of psy and neoliberal productivity and consumption standards—provides not only a possible manner of experiencing a discontent-turned-disease, as well as it delineates the 'exclusion' of modes of suffering from its grammar. Anxiety, in the shift in diagnosis observed since the 1980s, turns into a 'stranger'. The initial mass-pathologising of anxiety, followed by its breaking down into specific categories and diagnostic 'submission' to depression, as well as its 'management' through medication, accompany a cultural arrangement that is also observable outside of the clinic.

## Wellness or Hellness

An individualist concept of 'wellbeing' has permeated neoliberal times as our attitudes towards 'being not well' reflect the logic of quantification, categorisation and, ultimately, financialisation of late-capitalist ideology. Such an arrangement of 'wellbeing' extrapolates Foucault's account of modern governmentality as developed since the late eighteenth century under the paradigm of interiority and self-reference that permitted biopolitical subjectivation and towards which psychoanalysis is also allegedly a contributor (Foucault, 2004). The effort to 'feel good' in one's body is, in the contemporary context, also framed by the disciplinary and controlling assumption of the totality of conscious speech as promoter of attitude and behavioural changes—an assumption heavily questioned by psychoanalysis, which relies, on the contrary, precisely on the potential of representational lacunae, or gaps in language, which constitute the unconscious (Lacan, [1960] 2006). Freud taught us to take symbolisation and narrative with a 'pinch of salt', being more concerned with what lies underneath a clinical complaint. In current wellbeing discourse, 'mind and body' are articulated in such a manner that digital apps, checklists, as well as medication and even some 'yoga pants' have become the vocabulary to address bodies that are not 'balanced enough' and in need of management. All the while Big Pharma and the trillions of dollars-worth 'wellness industry' revel in profits (Cederström & Spicer, 2016; Reaney, 2014).

Alongside the solutions offered by Big Pharma, therapeutic practices based on self-monitoring, thinking 'positive' and setting clear 'goals' such as Cognitive Behavioural Therapy (CBT) and Positive Psychology have thrived under the logic of isolating symptoms and de-politicising suffering (Scull, 2019; Binkley, 2011). Currently, in the United Kingdom, guidelines for treating General Anxiety Disorder (GAD) promote the use of SSRI drugs as well as self-monitoring and individual or group self-help based on the principles of CBT (NICE, 2011). For Pilgrim (2008), "these socially mute technologies risk individualising distress and disconnecting it from its biographical and social origins" (Pilgrim, 2008, p. 258), promising, however, a 'quicker fix'. Argued as being a more 'effective' or simply put, 'cheaper' and easy to measure approach to therapy than long-term psychotherapy, CBT has been part of the NHS since the New Labour government of Tony Blair, promoted by his advisor from the London School of Economics, Richard Layard (Layard & Clark, 2014). The notions of 'efficiency' and 'productivity' unfold both in terms of governmental spending and of a mode of management of the self that delineates a problem based on the patient's complaint and works towards a clear goal that involves 'thinking and behaving' differently in order to rid oneself of an unwanted symptom (Pilgrim, 2008). In other words, "Cognitive-Behaviour Therapy (CBT) is based on the claim that the cause of distress lies in the individual's maladaptive thinking, or cognitive processes" (Proctor, 2008, p. 233).

In October 2007, the BBC (2007) reported on the announcement of increased funds for CBT which would widen the access to 'talking therapies' across the UK. It reads: "Health Secretary Alan Johnson said by 2010, £170 m a year would be spent—allowing 900,000 more people to be treated using psychological therapies. These are just as effective as drugs, says the National Institute of Health and Clinical Excellence. The plan will pay for itself as people return to work and stop needing benefits, an expert said". The discourse is remarkably centred around an economic argument for such investment in Mental Health treatment via CBT. Not surprisingly, its wide implementation in public mental health in the UK is a 'win-win' situation, except that it reinforces the isolation of symptoms and of the individual and one's competence in just 'acting' and 'changing' one's own patterns that are causing suffering. Such suffering is often costly to the state and, under this logic, should be 'easily' and strategically dealt with.

Beck and Ellis, the founders of CBT in the United States, were concerned with efficiency, avoiding the time consuming psychodynamic treatment, accordingly, their "primary interest was not about researching ordinary cognitive functioning (the norm in academic departments of psychology during the 1980s) but was about altering dysfunctional conduct" (Pilgrim, 2008, p. 251). Beck's Depression and Anxiety Inventories (BDI and BAI, respectively), specifically, are clinical tools that comprise 21-point checklist of surface symptoms that can be tackled in about ten minutes, not including any social, political, environmental or contextual factor for diagnosis of depression or anxiety. BDI and BAI, in their current formats, are widely used in primary care. It is not surprising that in the UK, unemployed people were offered CBT therapy "to help put Britain back to work" (Stratton, 2009).

As a paradox, yet reflecting the logic of such a therapeutic approach, governments, corporations and independent institutions have been investing in measuring 'happiness' exponentially in recent years, despite data on soaring inequality, precarity and mental health issues under austerity that circulate in the press (Segal, 2017). Economic problems and economic solutions to increase 'happiness' naturalise the paradigm of human capital even further, departing from a privatisation of suffering towards self-productivity management. Layard himself publishes his own *Happiness* book in 2005. 'Happiness' or 'well-being' seems secondary in such measuring policies once questions such as "what are these 'sufferings' telling us" are, if not ignored, bypassed by productivity metaphors. Cederström and Spicer comment on the rise of 'happiness officer' jobs and 'wellness contracts' in corporate institutions and universities, which are turning 'being happy' compulsory (Cederström & Spicer, 2016). 'Happiness pulses' and 'happy city' projects also echo such 'happiness is the new black' trend that leaves precisely the 'meaning' of what is considered as 'happy' out of the debate, as seen in a number of academic and theoretical critiques of the neoliberal 'culture of happiness' (Ahmed, 2010; Binkley, 2014; Davies, 2015; Cederström & Spicer, 2016; Segal, 2017). Overall the 'push to happiness' is grounded in Positive Psychology, a strand in the field of psy that aims at providing a 'management'-based system of achieving 'happiness' and that has been increasingly popularised in the twenty-first century. Utilising what is promoted as 'the most current techniques of psychological treatment' (Binkley, 2011, p. 373) this approach takes psychology away from the constant focus on 'negative' affects and preaches the regime for achieving a desired state of happiness. The founders of Positive Psychology are Martin Seligman and Mihaly Csikszentmihalyi, whose works had been focusing on adaptive behaviour and depression and the popular concept of 'flow' (present in many guides to Mindfulness, and meaning a total immersion and focus in one activity such as exercises, crafts, etc.), respectively (Binkley, 2014). The pair met in 1997 and, as Seligman was elected to the prestigious post of president of the American Psychological Association, they secured significant research funding across the USA, the UK and beyond for their work on popularising literature, tools, courses and guides (Binkley, 2014). Their work on Positive Psychology is presented on the back of their identification of 'Positive Personal Traits' such as 'optimism', 'courage', 'faith', 'work ethic' and so on as factors that lead to 'great' mental health. Their project envisaged that 'fostering excellence' should be the job of psychology as a whole in order to 'prevent' mental illness, in their words, as even 'normal' people need examples of positivity, as 'building optimism' can 'prevent depression' (Seligman & Csikszentmihalyi, 2000, p. 12).

In psychoanalytic terms, wellness culture presupposes an ideal-self, an Imaginary body, in the Lacanian sense of the term, towards which all such fantasies of an ideal state of plenitude and control are projected. In this conceptualisation, if we consider the promises of an ideal, purified and efficient self present in such discourses of consumption, there is a type of 'collective' fantasy being composed, and fantasies can only but leave something hanging out of them, something that will not fit into the frame of this projected ideal of selfhood. In a Lacanian view of this relation to fantasy, the cyclical attempt at fulfilling a fantasy and embodying an ideal that is impossible to ever be attained will open space for a failure, and this very failure will make way for anxiety. This opens up to a paradoxical cycle. On one hand there is the ubiquitous invocations for an individual 'work' on one's wellbeing, which passes through for example mass medicalisation, to Positive Psychology all the way into wellness trends. On the other hand, we can see these discourses promoting an 'easily-reachable' type of ideal wellbeing or ideal 'tuning' of the body and mind. However, by understanding this 'ideal' as a fantasy—one that leaves the subject to face the impossibility of ever feeling so 'good'—we can see this 'fantasy of control' opening the way to anxiety and then more anxiety. Therefore, it might be possible to trace a seemingly paradoxical cycle in which the subject is caught: from discontent to wellness; from such recourse to failing to feel as good as promised; from there to more anxiety and then back over to another wellness tool, maybe another medication or a different diet this time. Metaphorically, wellness can easily become *hellness*.

The discourses of 'management of the self' present in all these spheres—from diagnosis, to treatment and consumption—also reveal a typical characteristic of neoliberal capitalism: a constant praise and calculation of the 'individual' that at the same time leaves no space for the 'singular'. That is, the very promotion of a 'fit-efficient-pure-controlled' model for consumption or as goal and standard in mental health care presupposes that this ideal operates as a model that would work for 'everyone', cancelling or at least limiting the possibilities of singular potentialities, unique to each subject. The diagnostic-culture of our times, considering diagnosis and the promotion of wellbeing under such logic, reinforces, paradoxically, a state of constant anxiety that echoes a somewhat subjective precarity that anchors the mode of governance of contemporary capitalism. It comes to no surprise that by the end of 2020, according to *The Guardian*, the anxiety toll of Covid-19 saw 6 million new prescriptions of antidepressants in the UK only from July to September, 2020; and an overall spending of £139 million in antidepressants in 2020; £113 millions of which were in the SSRI Sertraline alone (Rabeea et al., 2021). Meanwhile, the NHS reported a drop in 235,000 referrals for talking therapy in the first semester of 2020 (Duncan & Marsh, 2021). One of or the biggest health crisis of a generation is, as we can see, tackled at the individual level by pills promoted through the serotogenic imbalance discourse (or, the premise that one's 'brain' does not produce correct amount of serotonin), rather than by exploring the nuanced distress of this crisis (which is also ecological and political) singularly and in context.

## Estranged from Anxiety: Modulation and Wellbeing

What the assemblage of wellness, psychiatric diagnosis, medicalisation of psychic experience and ultimately quantification of affect reveal is an affective-politics that accounts for body and psyche in a particular mode of alienation. Under the current affective-politics we can identify pharmacological corporations and governmentality replicating a modern scientific view of the body: described, divided, quantified and qualified. However, the demands for taming affective experiences are coupled with mechanisms of consumption and identification that result in postmodern technologies of subjectivity. This double-alienation that entails a colonisation of affect seen through the trail of anxiety is interestingly elucidated in Deleuze's mapping of the birth of the *dividual* (1992). Whilst Foucault delineates the modern individual as a locus of reproduction of a disciplinary society based in exclusions and division that took shape during the eighteenth and nineteenth centuries, Deleuze proposes that this modern individual has been further reduced into a *dividual*, the locus of reproduction of the society of control—one not based on exclusion, but based on identification, participation and endless quantification (Dosse, 2016). The shift into what he calls a society of control encompasses a transformation of 'molds' into 'modulations' of subjective production (Deleuze, 1992), as I will move into elaborating next. When thinking the trail of anxiety through this prism we can find concomitant 'mold' and 'modulation'-like qualities of the current psy-discourse. This particular encounter of *dispositifs* is precisely what qualifies the current affective-politics.

Wellbeing and governance have not become connected only in the last decades. On the contrary, it is an old modern alliance as it was particularly elaborated by Foucault in '*The Birth of Biopolitics*' lecture series from 1978 to 1979. In these lectures, he points to the fact that, 'wellbeing' is a term that emerged in the eighteenth century as a 'symbol' of state power in its full effectiveness, thus, having been crucial in ideological control and the mechanisms of biopower since the dawn of modernity (Foucault, 2008a, 2008b). Social regulation through the care of the body is, under this prism, bound to capitalism as the refinement of 'life-sciences' is historically linked to what Foucault calls the 'liberal art of governing' (Lazzarato, 2013). Deleuze calls such *dispositifs* 'molds' (1992) and defines their logic as follows:

> The disciplinary societies have two poles: the signature that designates the individual, and the number or administrative numeration that indicates his or her position within a mass. This is because the disciplines never saw any incompatibility between these two, and because at the same time power individualises and masses together, that is, constitutes those over whom it exercises power into a body and molds the individuality of each member of that body. (Deleuze, 1992, p. 5)

In this sense, the project of the DSM as a whole could be compared to a 'mold' as it offers a homogenisation of whatever heterogeneity is present in the forms of discontent and suffering experienced in society. The DSM and the *raison d'être* of efforts in categorising and identifying aetiological frames for mental illness marked across the field of psy provide a 'name', a 'number' and a 'diagnosis' through which an individual can be 'positioned within a mass'. Such reduction of the multiplicity in manners of suffering to the same common 'grammar' and particularly 'normative' gramma. It generates an imposition of uniformity on symptoms based on a contemporary Western paradigm of pathology, resulting in a "neutralization of the critical potential that psychological symptoms bring to the understanding of a determined social context, as the role that symptoms have always played" (Dunker, 2015, p. 35). In other words, psychiatry emerges as a discourse of 'morality', distinguishing what 'normal' and desirable look like (Birman, 1978). Furthermore, there is also a neutralisation of the potential to produce new modalities of the social bond carried by 'discontents' in their singularity and multiplicity. Another 'mold'-like characteristic of the diagnostic-culture inaugurated in the 1980s can be observed in its biological, or organicist, traits that reduce discontent to sensorial pain and suffering, thereby reducing the subject to the 'fleshy' body.

In the 'modulation' of 'societies of control' that unfold in the twentieth century, the picture is slightly more complex yet not too dissimilar. Deleuze describes the shift as follows:

> In the societies of control, on the other hand, what is important is no longer either a signature or a number, but a code: the code is a password, while on the other hand the disciplinary societies are regulated by watchwords (as much from the point of view of integration as from that of resistance). The numerical language of control is made of codes that mark access to information, or reject it. We no longer find ourselves dealing with the mass/individual pair. Individuals have become 'dividuals', and masses, samples, data, markets, or 'banks'. (Deleuze, 1992, p. 5)

One manner of illustrating what Deleuze means by 'modulated dividuals' is the 'quantified self' phenomenon in relation to wellbeing. Noting that people usually refuse or at least do not collaborate with reporting on their mental health for research, Davies (2015) cites the digital platforms and devices operated by companies such as Google or Nike through which users are 'happily' willing to offer details, "and report on various aspects of their private lives—from their diets, to their moods, to their sex lives" (Davies, 2015, p. 221). Such 'enthusiasm for self-surveillance' is welcomed by corporations that are now investing in novel health and fitness products (e.g. Fitbit, Strava or Apple Watch) that "can be sold alongside quantified self apps, which will allow individuals to make constant reports of their behaviour (such as jogging), generating new data sets for the company in the process" (Davies, 2015, p. 221). Data thus becomes a 'password' and offers recognition in the digitally informed social sphere. At the same time, each tap, each word, each interaction is translated into chunks of big-data that, in its turn, bounces back in the form of targeted advertising operated through algorithms on the web.

In this sense, the alliance between the DSM-model and the pharmaceutical industry, which relies heavily on marketing, echoes the 'modulation' of experience. Consumption of medication becomes the 'password' and the body, the fleshy body, is modulated as 'medication adjustments' operate by isolating parts and functions of the body, creating "artificial zones of contention, excitation, anaesthesia and separation that work as protective walls against discontent and zones of exception against suffering" (Dunker, 2015, p. 28). 'Dividuality' and the modus operandi of the society of control are evidenced in the new function of psychopathological diagnosis under the current diagnostic-culture. Instead of representing a force of exclusion from social life, as the asylum did for example, the consumption of medication(s) justified by a systematic categorisation of affects, symptoms and manners of suffering and being provide, as a modulating mapping of the fleshy body, a type of 'fantasy' of recognition in the model of a 'password'. As Dunker summarises, "if previously the psychopathological diagnosis could mean a terrifying and at times irreversible inclusion in the juridical-hospital frame or moral-educational exclusion, now it seems to have become a powerful and disseminated means of determination and recognition, if not even a means of destitution of the responsibility of a subject" (Dunker, 2015, p. 33). A diagnosis can, under the paradigm of productivity, offer a form of relief from such a burden.

Deleuze, however, leaves an impression that in the present time, Foucault's 'disciplinary societies' were being substituted by this new order of control, as if one followed the other. This 'misunderstanding' is, as defended by Gerald Raunig, in part due to the nature of Deleuze's text itself (Raunig, 2009). 'Postscript on Societies of Control', the text, is extremely short, barely reaching five pages of length, and written in a very poetic—and apocalyptic, if one may add—style. What Raunig stresses is that 'modulation' "is the name of this merging of discipline society and control society: as the aspects of discipline and control are always to be seen as intertwined" (Raunig, 2009). Thus, the seeming linearity of temporal sequence open for interpretation in the original text is one of its 'weaknesses'. Deleuze's text reads as follows:

> But everyone knows that these institutions are finished, whatever the length of their expiration periods. It's only a matter of administering their last rites and of keeping people employed until the last installation of the new forces knocking at the door. These are the societies of control, which are in the process of replacing the disciplinary societies. (Deleuze, 1992, p. 4)

Indeed, this passage evokes a temporal linearity that does not translate in the shifts from enclosed confinement of institutions towards an open and multiple form of ever-changing casts. Rather, as Raunig points out, what we experience in the twenty-first century and what characterises modulation is "an accumulation of both aspects" (Raunig, 2009), a simultaneous presence of both models, intertwined and intercalating. Social subjugation and 'forced adaptation'—the hetero into homogeneous, from mass to individual—accompany the "modes of self-government in a totally transparent, open milieu, and discipline through personal surveillance and punishment couples with the liberal visage of control as voluntary self-control" (Raunig, 2009) that 'modulates' a 'dividual'.

The encounter of modulating-molds and of *dispositifs* of subjective production and reproduction found in tracing the trail of anxiety in mainstream psychiatric discourses allows us to elucidate, even if a little, the current arrangements of colonisation of psychic experience and affective life. Given this cartography of anxiety and the place of an anxious *dividual* in it, we can ask whether the *dividual* can speak. If anxiety is the compass that can lead us to a world beyond the veils of fantasies, if it can push novel arrangements of the social bond, it seems that an anxious *dividual* is left at the cliff-edge of an existential abyss that only grows deeper at the hands of hegemonic psy-discourses.

The antagonism present in this ideological organisation of a 'society of control' is interestingly situated in the body of the 'anxious dividual' of the contemporary and revealed in the relation of a 'modulating estrangement' to one's anxiety. The system of diagnosis and management of the body and its affects, whilst crossed by ideological power, produce an 'impossibility' towards living with one's anxiety. Anxiety travels from a mass-pathologised status to an ideology-informed disappearance within the diagnostic system and makes a return in the form of a highly medicalised and isolated symptom. The ever-expanding DSM editions and the 'checklist' approach in use operate as 'molding watchwords'. At the same time, the consumption discourse of care of the body and mind, present in wellness culture, elevates the treatment framework of elimination and management of anxiety via the care of the body to the function of what Deleuze calls a 'modulating password'. Such discourses, in and outside of the clinic, are *dividualising*, as within their modus operandi there is no space left for the possibility of singularity. Whilst they offer a series of 'fixing tools' centred on the body, these discourses presuppose, at the same time, a 'same' form of suffering that should be common to all *dividuals* they are addressing with their modulating 'grammar'. In such a quantifying culture, the subject is locked out of the possibility of seeing what is beyond the lifting of curtains of fantasy, as Freud and Lacan proposed (Verhaeghe, 2014). The management of anxiety 'away' from one's body is, therefore, the logic of the relation of 'estrangement' we will move into questioning, within a psychoanalytic approach.

The drive, the unconscious and the '*transindividual*' aspects of psychic life and the self are what set psychoanalytic theory and practice aside from other discourses of mental health and wellbeing that are ideologically divergent within the field of the broad psychological discourses of the contemporary context. Such dividing differences are evidenced in the understanding of the symptom and, by consequence, of suffering and the mind-body riddle. A key difference between, for example, Cognitive-Behavioural Therapy and psychoanalysis would be the more simplistic cause and effect relation in the former, which is based on clinical techniques proposed by Ellis and Beck and successors in the United States from the 1960s onwards, where a thought becomes a recurrent 'automatic' cognitive route leading to specific behaviours and patterns of feeling (Rose, 2018). Beyond this direct causality, what becomes definitive in the divide between these approaches is the reliance on a 'knowing' and conscious awareness in the process of offering a narrative of oneself, that meaning, a clinical reliance on the patient bringing a problem and that being accepted or assumed as the actual 'problem', or all there is to it, usually leading to a change in behaviour in order to ease, deal or in a more unfortunate case scenario simply aim at getting rid of such a 'problem'. With the *transindividual* unconscious at work and the drive as cornerstones of psychic life, psychoanalysis complicates such views of re-educating consciously one's thoughts and behaviours—as Positive Psychology assumes—simply because a psychoanalytic narrative of oneself implies a very powerful not-knowing and its reverberations, being thus a challenge or impossibility to the project of measuring and categorising of evidence-based experimental psychological traditions.

Anxiety is understood in psychoanalytic literature, from the Freudian and Lacanian orientation, as the affect of excess. Instead of isolating anxiety by turning it into a symptom or disorder and systematically attempting to 'eliminate' one's anxiety, psychoanalysis listens to anxiety and to what it may be possibly telling of the positioning of the subject in question in relation to their experience. However, the tools of interpretation, the social and subjective models of psychoanalysis and, further, psychoanalysis' very onto-epistemic foundations enclose anxiety to an 'abyss within', as I will move into arguing next. A modern humanist, patriarchal and colonial inheritance still permeates both theory and praxis. In our cartography, our goal is to think beyond such hauntings in the clinic of anxiety.

## References

ADAA. (2021). Understanding Anxiety: Facts and Statistics. [Online]. https://adaa.org/about-adaa/press-room/facts-statistics

Ahmed, S. (2010). *The Promise of Happiness*. Duke University Press.

BBC. (2007, October 10). More Funds for Talking Therapies. *BBC* [Online]. http://news.bbc.co.uk/1/hi/health/7037400.stm
Binkley, S. (2011). Happiness, Positive Psychology and the Program of Neoliberal Governmentality. *Subjectivity, 4*(4), 371–394.
Binkley, S. (2014). *Happiness as Enterprise: An Essay on Neoliberal Life*. State University of New York Press.
Birman, J. (1978). *A Psiquiatria como discurso da moralidade*. Graal.
Callard, F. (2014). Psychiatric Diagnosis: The Indispensability of Ambivalence. *Journal of Medical Ethics, 40*, 526–530.
Callard, F. (2016). The Intimate Geographies of Panic Disorder: Parsing Anxiety Through Psychopharmacological Dissection. *OSIRIS, 31*, 203–226.
Campbell, D. (2017, June 29). NHS Prescribed Record Number of Antidepressants Last Year. *The Guardian* [Online]. https://www.theguardian.com/society/2017/jun/29/nhs-prescribed-record-number-of-antidepressants-last-year
Cederström, C., & Spicer, A. (2016). *The Wellness Syndrome*. Polity.
Cohen, B. (2016). *Psychiatric Hegemony: A Marxist Theory of Mental Illness*. Palgrave Macmillan.
Cooke, R. (2013, September 15). Living with Anxiety: Britain's Silent Epidemic. *The Guardian* [Online]. https://www.theguardian.com/society/2013/sep/15/anxiety-epidemic-gripping-britain
Crocq, M. A. (2015). A History of Anxiety: From Hippocrates to DSM. *Dialogues in Clinical Neuroscience, 17*(3), 319–325.
Crocq, M. A. (2017). The history of generalised anxiety disorder as a diagnostic category. *Dialogues in Clinical Neuroscience, 19*(2), 107–116.
Davies, W. (2015). *The Happiness Industry: How the Government and Big Business Sold Us Well-Being*. Verso.
Deleuze, G. (1992). Postscript on Societies of Control. *October, 59*, 3–7.
Dosse, F. (2016). Deleuze and Foucault: A Philosophical Friendship. In N. Morar, T. Nail, & D. Smith (Eds.), *Between Deleuze and Foucault*. Edinburgh University Press.
Duncan, P., & Marsh, S. (2021, January 1). Antidepressant Use in England Soars as Pandemic Cuts Counselling Access. *The Guardian* [Online]. https://www.theguardian.com/society/2021/jan/01/covid-antidepressant-use-at-all-time-high-as-access-to-counselling-in-england-plunges
Dunker, C. (2015). *Mal-Estar, Sofrimento e Sintoma*. Boitempo Editorial.
Ehrenberg, A. (2009). *The Weariness of the Self. Diagnosing the History of Depression in the Contemporary Age*. McGill-Queen University Press.

Foucault, M. (1982). The Subject and Power. *Critical Inquiry, 8*(4, Summer), 777–795.
Foucault, M. (2004). *Abnormal: Lectures at the Collège de France, 1974-1975*. Palgrave Macmillan.
Foucault, M. (2008a). *The Birth of Biopolitics: Lectures at The Collège de France 1978-79*. Palgrave Macmillan.
Foucault, M. (2008b). *Mental Illness and Psychology*. University of California Press.
Guéry, F., & Deleule, D. (2014). *The Productive Body*. Zero Books.
Harrington, A. (2019). *Mind Fixers: Psychiatry's Troubled Search for the Biology of Mental Illness*. W.W. Norton & Company.
Herzberg, D. (2009). *Happy Pills in America: From Miltown to Prozac*. Johns Hopkins University Press.
Horwitz, A. (2010). How an Age of Anxiety Became an Age of Depression. *The Milbank Quarterly, 88*(1), 112–138.
Horwitz, A. (2013). *Anxiety: A Short History*. The Johns Hopkins University Press.
Horwitz, A., & Wakefield, J. (2012). *All We Have to Fear. Psychiatry's Transformation of Natural Anxieties into Mental Disorders*. Oxford.
Kehl, M. R. (2015). *O tempo e o Cão. A atualidade das depressões*. Editora Boitempo.
Lacan, J. (1960). The Subversion of the Subject and the Dialectic of Desire in the Freudian Unconscious. In *Écrits:* The First Complete Edition in English (2006) [Trans. B. Fink]. W.W. Norton and Company.
Layard, R. (2005). *Happiness: Lessons from a New Science*. Penguin.
Layard, R., & Clark, D. M. (2014). *Thrive: The Power of Evidence-Based Psychological Therapies*. Penguin.
Lazzarato, M. (2013). Governmentality in the Current Crisis. *Generation Online* [Online]. http://www.generation-online.org/p/fp_lazzarato7.htm
Metzl, J. (2003). *Prozac on the Couch: Prescribing Gender in the Era of Wonder Drugs*. Duke University Press.
Mojtabai, R., & Olfson, M. (2008). National Patterns in Antidepressant Treatment by Psychiatrists and General Medical Providers: Results from the National Comorbidity Survey Replication. *Journal of Clinical Psychiatry, 69*, 1064–1074.
NICE. (2011). National Institute for Health Care Excellence: Principles of Care for People with Generalised Anxiety Disorder. [Online]. https://www.nice.org.uk/guidance/cg113/chapter/1-Guidance#principles-of-care-for-people-with-generalised-anxiety-disorder-gad
NIHM. (2021). Any Anxiety Disorder. [Online]. https://www.nimh.nih.gov/health/statistics/prevalence/any-anxiety-disorder-among-adults.shtml

ONS. (2018). Methodology: Surveys Using the 4 Office for National Statistics Personal Well-being Questions. [Online]. https://www.ons.gov.uk/peoplepopulationandcommunity/wellbeing/methodologies/surveysusingthe4officefornationalstatisticspersonalwellbeingquestions

ONS. (2020). Personal and Economic Well-being in Great Britain: May 2020. [Online]. https://www.ons.gov.uk/peoplepopulationandcommunity/wellbeing/bulletins/personalandeconomicwellbeingintheuk/may2020#elevated-levels-of-anxiety

Palmary, I., & Barnes, B. (2015). Critical Psychology in Africa. The Impossible Task. In I. Parker (Ed.), *Handbook of Critical Psychology*. Routledge.

Pinel, P. (1806). *A Treatise on Insanity*. Messers Cadell & Davies.

Pilgrim, D. (2008). Reading 'Happiness': CBT and the Layard Thesis. *European Journal of Psychotherapy and Counselling, 10*(3), 247–260.

Proctor, G. (2008). CBT: The Obscuring of Power in the Name of Science. *European Journal of Psychotherapy and Counselling, 10*(3), 231–245.

Rabeea, S. A., Merchant, H. A., Khan, M. U., et al. (2021). Surging Trends in Prescriptions and Costs of Antidepressants in England Amid COVID-19. *DARU Journal of Pharmaceutical Sciences, 29*, 217–221.

Raunig, G. (2009, August). In Modulation Mode: Factories of Knowledge. *Transversal* [Online]. http://eipcp.net/transversal/0809/raunig/en

Reaney, P. (2014, October 1). Global Spa, Wellness Industry Estimated at $3.4trillion: Report. *Reuters* [Online]. http://uk.reuters.com/article/us-life-wellness-idUKKCN0HP2OK20140930

Rose, N. (1996). *Inventing Ourselves. Psychology, Power and Personhood*. Cambridge University Press.

Rose, N. (2006). Disorders Without Borders? The Expanding Scope of Psychiatric Practice. *BioSocieties, 1*, 465–484.

Rose, N. (2007). *The Politics of Life Itself – Biomedicine, Power, and Subjectivity. In the Twenty-First Century*. Princeton University Press.

Rose, N. (2018). *Our Psychiatric Future: The Politics of Mental Health*. Polity Press.

Sadowsky, J. (2021). *The Empire of Depression. A New History*. Polity.

Scull, A. (2019). *Psychiatry and Its Discontents*. University of California Press.

Segal, L. (2017). *Radical Happiness. Moments of Collective Joy*. Verso.

Seligman, M., & Csikszentmihalyi, M. (2000). Positive Psychology: An Introduction. *American Psychologist, 55*, 5–14.

Sharma, R. (2020, May 4). Coronavirus and Mental Health: Pharmacists Are Struggling to Source Antidepressants, After a Rise in Demand During Lockdown. *iNews* [Online]. https://inews.co.uk/news/health/

mental-health-coronavirus-antidepressants-medication-supplies-uk-lockdown-rise-demand-2842273

Shorter, E. (2005). *A Historical Dictionary of Psychiatry*. Oxford University Press.

Shorter, E. (2009). *Before Prozac: The Troubled History of Mood Disorders in Psychiatry*. Oxford University Press.

Sprengnether, M. (1995). Mourning Freud. In S. Frosh & A. Elliot (Eds.), *Psychoanalysis in Contexts. Paths Between Theory and Modern Culture*. Routledge.

Stratton, A. (2009, December 4). Jobless to Be Offered 'talking treatment' to Help Put Britain Back to Work. *The Guardian* [Online]. https://www.theguardian.com/society/2009/dec/04/jobless-therapy-talking-cbt-unemployment

Vanheule, S. (2014). *Diagnosis and the DSM: A Critical Review*. Palgrave Macmillan.

Verhaeghe, P. (2008). *On Being Normal and Other Disorders. A Manual for Clinical Psychodiagnostics*. Karnac.

Verhaeghe, P. (2014). *What About Me? The Struggle for Identity in a Market-based Society*. Scribe.

Whitaker, R. (2010). *Anatomy of an Epidemic: Magic Bullets, Psychiatric Drugs, and the Astonishing Rise of Mental Illness in America*. Crown Publisher-Random House.

# 4

# Abysses and Horizons: Why Psychoanalysis?

The field of psy, as we have seen in these initial meanders and incursions, is drenched in subjective ideals of cure, treatment, pathology and normality. The ideological compass orienting the function of the clinic reveals, accordingly, political consequences implied in epistemological and ontological foundations of clinical praxis. As Nikolas Rose puts it, "the idea of the norm, as it came into use in the late nineteenth century, linked together the ideas of statistical normality, social normality and medical normality: the norm was the average, the desirable, the healthy, the ideal and so forth" (Rose, 2018, p. 9). In this sense, "normality—of what it is to be normal, to think of oneself as normal, to be considered as normal by others—leads to a set of rather profound questions" (Rose, 2018, p. 9). As such, the pathologisation of anxiety and the enquiry over what anxiety is all about, what it is telling us and what are the grounds of its emergence have meet question of 'what can anxiety do?'. Now, we look into the question of what psychoanalysis can offer to the treatment of anxiety and why this is a path still worth pursuing, whilst considering the many 'dividualising' aspects of the psychoanalytic discourse itself.

The matter of the ideological foundations of treatment in the field of psy is dealt with philosophically with this horizon of situating anxiety as 'vibration', orienting this effort in relation to the limits of 'being' and


A. C. Minozzo, *Anxiety as Vibration*, Studies in the Psychosocial,
https://doi.org/10.1007/978-3-031-62856-6_4

possibilities of 'becoming' in the experience of anxiety. To do so, we are investigating the psychoanalytic unconscious in the understanding of the affect of anxiety, which leads us to a point of 'excess', and this is what we will tour in more detail through a discussion on the foundations of 'negativity' in psychoanalysis of the Freudian and Lacanian orientations. An increased focus on biological, behavioural and individualised aspects of psychological distress in contemporary understandings of anxiety becomes evident. In psychoanalysis, conversely, unconscious, relational and contextual elements frame distress and symptoms.

## Anxiety and Psychoanalysis, Excesses

The manner in which psychiatry deals with psychic suffering through the twentieth century can be characterised as a 'descriptive psychopathology' (Berrios, 1996). Biology and individual causality are at the heart of the efforts of the DSM-III, IV and V (Rose, 2018), where the affect of anxiety is divided, listed and pathologised accordingly. This debate involves complex philosophical and ideological assumptions that permeate wider discourses in psychiatry, psychologies and psychoanalysis that meet precisely at the complicated, yet often oversimplified, definition of what is normal and what is pathological in affective life. In other words, the riddle of quantifying and qualifying 'how much anxiety is too much?' is the backbone of a contemporary *dividual, estranged from anxiety*.

Eighteenth- and early-nineteenth century medical literature discussed what were considered both 'subjective' (fear, phobia, etc.) and 'objective' (digestive, respiratory, etc.) aspects of what was later combined into the understanding of 'anxiety' disorders or symptoms as unrelated phenomena that were formative of other illnesses and of madness. In other words, "by the mid-nineteenth century, the term anxiety was used in medical writings to describe a mental state that fell within the range of normal human experiences but was able to cause or lead to disease, including insanity" (Berrios, 1996, p. 266). Bodily and psychological experiences were, therefore, bound in anxiety. Yet, it was only in the later decades of the nineteenth century that the prominence of a 'nervous' system, or a ganglionar system, gave rise to an understanding of anxiety as having something to do with an excessive production of some sort from within the body and a link with perception—or what was being sensed from outside. This focus on the nerves and neurology in the works of physicians such as Xavier Bichat, Bénédict Morel and chiefly George Miller Beard (Shorter, 2005) both in the USA and in Europe would see the diagnosis of 'neurasthenia' grow in popularity, containing symptoms of what we would now understand as anxiety or even an anxiety or panic attack (Berrios, 1996). In the context of such diagnoses of a 'weakness of the nerves' and of the social and medical enigma of hysteria, psychoanalysis emerges as a clinical approach that accounted for the unconscious traces and logics at the heart of symptoms. The psychoanalytic emphasis on anxiety can be found in a very early theoretical proposition written by Freud, 'On The Grounds for Detaching a Particular Syndrome From Neurasthenia Under The Description "Anxiety Neurosis"' (1894). Anxiety neurosis was here being called as such "because all its components can be grouped round the chief symptom of anxiety, because each one of them has a definite relationship to anxiety" (Freud, 1894, p. 91). Freud, in this paper, recognises the potential similarities in diagnosis of cases of neurasthenia and anxiety neurosis, but he moves on to clarifying the difference between the two as lying precisely in the specific sexual origins of anxiety neurosis—the sexual can be interpreted with a more contemporary inflection as libidinal or concerning what Lacan names *jouissance*, an enjoyment beyond the scope of the subject.

Freud also defends that the psychoanalytic method is the only one capable of providing in-depth enough interpretations which not only proved his theory of anxiety neurosis right but also unveiled symptoms. He writes "it is impossible to pursue an aetiological investigation based on anamneses if we accept those anamneses as the patients present them, or are content with what they are willing to volunteer" (Freud, 1895, p. 129).[1] In other words, we cannot take presented symptoms or narra-

[1] It is worth mentioning how this statement seemingly leaves the power of being the 'archaeologist' of the mind and the holder of knowledge on the side of the analyst, similarly to the logic of the prototypical models of diagnosis in psychiatry. Lacan displaces this position by considering the analyst the subject 'supposed to know' rather than the one who actually knows in the transference. *Co-poiesis* thus expands on being 'supposed to know' by encouraging a horizontal collaborative production in the clinic.

tives of complaints at face value, once they are not the 'full picture', once consciousness is not sufficient to depict the grounds of psychic suffering. The unconscious marks a division among methods, interpretations and treatments in the field of psy, wrapping symptoms around it.

In psychoanalysis, anxiety is defined as an affect, mobilising therefore 'body' and 'mind' equally. Anxiety "includes in the first place particular motor innervations or discharges and secondly certain feelings; the latter are of two kinds—perceptions of the motor actions that have occurred and the direct feelings of pleasure and unpleasure which, as we say, give the affect its keynote" (Freud, 1917, p. 395). In other words, the affect of anxiety situates the subject in relation to what is beyond oneself, stretching perception and feelings that are both bodily and psychological, of one's position in the world—challenging thus the dividualising foundations of mainstream psychiatric and psychological care. This move or encounter with an abyss-within or a horizon-beyond oneself is at the centre of the unsettling, overwhelming but also creative potential of this 'exceptional affect' that marks an appearance of what Lacan named the register of the Real (Soler, 2014). What makes anxiety really compelling also theoretically is how both Freud and Lacan have cast it as an affect of 'excess', as this close study of their work on anxiety in the next chapters will reveal. For Freud, as per his 1917 *Introductory Lecture* on anxiety, anxiety is an excessive affect that escapes the ego's attempts of repressing or representing a libidinal vicissitude—castration anxiety points thus to the threat an overwhelming libido poses to the ego, which in its turn acts as a psychic gatekeeper of stability in Freudian topology.

Post-Freudians, in particular Melanie Klein, interpret and modify Freud's topological model, which, after his publication of 'Beyond the Pleasure Principle', in 1919, and 'The Ego and the Id', in 1923, shifts his theories of anxiety to the workings of the Ego, Id and Super-Ego. Klein's work places anxiety at the centre of the psyche, with an idea that babies are born 'full' of this overwhelming intensity, which towards her later writings she saw as a manifestation of the death drive. In 'The Theory of Anxiety and Guilt' (1948), Klein writes: "My contention that anxiety originates in the fear of annihilation derives from experience accumulated in the analyses of young children" (Klein, [1948] 1988, p. 29). Anxiety, for her, is centrally connected to guilt, which, in turn, fuels the shift from an early paranoid-schizoid position, where "hatred and persecutory anxiety become attached to the frustrating (bad) breast, and love and reassurance to the gratifying (good) breast" (Klein, [1948] 1988, p. 34). Some states of transitory integration between the good and the bad part-objects give rise to a "synthesis between love and hatred [...] which gives rise to depressive anxiety" (Klein, [1948] 1988, p. 34). This transition towards the depressive position, where reparation becomes possible, is formative of the ego, which in development would be able to handle both what she called 'persecutory anxiety' and 'depressive anxiety', equipped with the necessary defence-mechanisms to experience both anxieties. In her words, such a mechanism is "the ego's capacity of evolving adequate defences against anxiety, i.e. the proportion of the strength of anxiety to the strength of the ego" (Klein, [1948] 1988, p. 40). Klein forged her own theory of anxiety, with much creativity; carving her original reading of the function of this affect, she writes: "An optimum in the interaction between libido and aggression implies that the anxiety arising from the perpetual activity of the death instinct, though never eliminated, is counteracted and kept at bay by the power of the life instinct" (Klein, [1948] 1988, p. 42). In Klein's clinical technique, and similarly in other Object Relational traditions that would follow in the twentieth century, the analyst works through the transference and countertransference envisaging offering a therapeutic reparation (Rustin, 2015) through introjections of qualities from the relation with the analyst and interpretations that act to uncover and symbolise unconscious phantasies.

Lacan was rather sceptical of the techniques employed by Klein in the clinic and the belief in the possibility of full-symbolisation of a phantasy, as well as of prospects of life under a strong and stable ego, as, to him, the ego, especially as it was formulated by the Ego-Analysts in the United States, pertained to the register of the Imaginary. The Imaginary in Lacan can be summarised as the function that offers coherence to the world 'outside' through the 'image', or the mirage of the subject. Its limits, the limits of this anchoring 'mirage' and 'subjective coherence', are particularly relevant to understanding anxiety, as in anxiety the fictional character of this subjective mirage becomes evident—or better, the mirage is under threat, the abyss comes near (Lacan, 1960). For Lacan, it is in anxiety that the Real makes an 'apparition', since "anxiety highlights how much of the subject is not captured by language, or how much is left over after the most exhaustive attempts to encapsulate or represent the subject in words" (Gallagher, 1996, p. 5). Because of its relation to the Real, anxiety points at a failure of fantasy, and this theoretical relation is developed in detail throughout Lacan's *Seminar X* on Anxiety, delivered between 1962 and 1963. Fantasy functions as a cover up for a fundamental 'structural fault' of the subject, and it fails to provide this efficient covering up in the moment of anxiety. This fact alone alludes to something beyond symbolisation, something that fails and in failing is unique to each subject that is evident in anxiety. In other words, the mirage of the subject is destabilised in anxiety. The curtain is lifted, a veil evaporates.

The psychoanalytic view of anxiety reiterates the psychoanalytic understanding of the symptom and diagnosis. This means that it goes against the logic of contemporary hegemonic discourses in psychology and psychiatry, in which anxiety is treated as a generator of 'disorders' in its own right or as an isolated symptom to be 'cured' or 'managed away'. For Lacan, as much as for Freud, anxiety is not 'the problem', let alone 'a problem to be eliminated' in the search of some 'cure'. What the trail of anxiety reveals to us in our psychosocial analysis of its journey in and out of the clinic, from the mid to late twentieth century until the current moment, is an affective-politics, or an affective domination, that steers the subject away from any possibility of living with their anxiety, their affects or conceiving life beyond the curtain or the veil of fantasy. Working with anxiety as an affect of 'excess', however, is not a conventional or unproblematic position psychoanalytically, especially when it touches the very onto-epistemic foundations of Freudian and Lacanian thought. And that is so in relation to the function of what frames such excess (fantasy, defences or Oedipal-identifications) in the model of subjectivity that informs a psy praxis.

## The Normal, the Pathological and the Unconscious

During the twentieth century, several scholars and practitioners have questioned psychiatric hegemony and the socio-political implications of 'normality'. From the works of Thomas Szasz and Erving Goffman in the United States, to David Cooper and R.D. Laing in Britain, as well as Robert Castel and Franco Basaglia in France and Italy, the myths and makings of mental illness have integrated what is understood as the (still polemic) field of critical psychiatry and psychology (Middleton & Moncrieff, 2019). In France, during the 1940s and 1950s, Georges Canguilhem was closely associated with the radical clinic of Saint-Alban, where Tosquelles, Jean Oury and Franz Fanon also lived and worked, taking Lacan's psychoanalytic 'return to Freud' into the institution and furthering its potencies in the treatment of psychoses (Robcis, 2021). Canguilhem (1991), in *On the Normal and the Pathological*, from 1943, what characterises a form of suffering that is 'enough of a problem' to be considered a 'pathology' appears always in contrast with an idea—or ideal—of normativity that frames the subject ideologically through ranking possibilities of recognition of such suffering. As such, and building from the movements of pathologising and diagnosing anxiety, we can agree that there is neither a 'normal' nor a 'pathological' in itself, rather, there are only these qualifications within the relation between an organism and the environment. Social context and the context produced by the qualifications generated by the psychologies (and in an ample manner, the psy-field) are crucial elements of any interpretation of 'suffering'. In short, what Canguilhem proposes is that the characterisation of what is to suffer 'normally' or not is a producer of this very suffering too. This ideological matter and its consequences have been examined in detail through the 'grammar' of anxiety. Still, if psychoanalysis is to offer anything different to this grammar, we must look at it closer and answer: why psychoanalysis as our road towards an anxiety as vibration?

In the essay 'What is Psychology?', from the late 1950s, Canguilhem adds a further layer to his critique of the 'sciences' of *psyche*, asserting that "it is inevitable that in presenting itself as the general theory of behaviour, psychology will incorporate some idea of Man. Hence, it is necessary that we allow philosophy to question psychology about where this idea comes from, and whether it may not be, ultimately, some philosophy" (Canguilhem, 2016, p. 202). We can unpack this problem in two different manners. First: the context producing and qualifying suffering as well as the ideological normativity implicated when assessing this suffering are not neutral. These initial points are fundamental to inquiring about this affect in a non-normative manner and asking what is the role of both diagnosis and cultural discourses in the contemporary understanding of anxiety. That is, how do diagnoses and culture produce our relation to this affect at an individual level? Second: there is an idea—and again, an ideal—of subjectivity predicted in the very object of psychology, and by being so, questions brought by philosophy (and critical theories, in general, including feminist, ecological and decolonial epistemologies) cannot be dismissed. In other words, psychology operates within an ontology epistemically situated, or an understanding of the subject bound within a scientific discourse. Therefore, if ever speaking of an 'anxious self' or 'anxious subject', it is necessary to make it clear what this notion of self in question is and how it is produced. This movement of contextualising the conditions of subjective production and reproduction is, in particular, one that permeates the psychosocial landscape.

In both elements of Canguilhem's critiques, there is something that sets psychoanalysis apart from other psychological practices, especially those in evidence in the present time (such as CBT, Positive Psychology and biological psychiatry). To follow this argument, we can return to Foucault (2008), who questions in *Mental Illness and Psychology* (from 1954) the limits between what is considered a 'pathology' of the organic/physical domain and the 'mental' or more subjective realm. These two realms are, in Freudian psychoanalysis, as Foucault sees it, worked through a complementary psyche-soma that extends beyond a simple or linear etiological 'cause and effect' relation. As an illustrative example we could think of the early texts on hysteria in *Studies on Hysteria*, in which psychological phenomena implicate the body and are implicated by the body enigmatically, rather than linearly. More clearly, in the Freudian notion of the *drive* (*pulsion*, *Trieb*, first mistranslated as 'instinct' into English), a complex interrelation of mind/body, without necessarily privileging any part over the other is at stake. As a contrast, an example of a cause/effect and a dualism between body/mind can be found in the organicist psychiatric discourse that attempts to locate suffering in the brain and treats mental 'malaise' through a rebalancing of chemical substances, natural or not to the human organism. Psychoanalysis, accordingly, sits in between the organic-medical discourse and a philosophical understanding of the self/subject that amplifies the understanding of a self beyond the physical body yet not transcending it completely. Psychoanalysis however moves over from a 'soul versus flesh' pre-modern narrative that nineteenth century psychology set as the line between religion and science (Guéry & Deleule, 2014). In psychoanalysis, materiality and discursivity are intertwined in a subject that is intrinsically political; therefore, suffering is never completely alienated from its context, neither is it totally absorbed by it. Suffering operates instead as this point of tension between the singular and the contextual.

To all psychologies, and to psychoanalysis too, and perhaps here being a different project than that of philosophy or of social sciences, questions of method or object are superseded by one matter that seems to have greater importance, that is of the clinical 'efficiency' or 'probity' in 'treating' a patient and their psychic suffering. Rather than a neat theory, psychologies and psychoanalysis, in the best case-scenarios, are grounded in the clinic. Canguilhem reminds us that to free itself from the 'unscientific' rancid aftertaste of being the 'science of the soul', "in 19th and 20th centuries, the psychology of reaction and behaviour thought it made itself independent by separating itself from all philosophy, that is to say, from the kind of speculation that looks for an idea of Man beyond the biological and sociological facts" (Canguilhem, 2016, p. 212). However, this system of verification of reality—let alone the classification of the possibilities of reality seen in the following diagnostic manuals for instance—led to an artificial doubling up of the reality of the 'classifier', or the psychologist, over the reality of the 'classified', the 'mentally ill' patient. As he puts it, the behavioural focus of the nineteenth and twentieth century—and even, we could propose, its contemporary twist in Cognitive-Behavioural Therapy—"could not prevent the recurrence of its results in the behaviour of those who obtain them" (Canguilhem, 2016, p. 212). In other words, the power relation established between the expert and the patient actualises diagnoses (Proctor, 2008)—echoing what Marcuse (1969) calls a 'corporealisation of the superego', or a symptomatic embodiment of authority. By separating itself from any 'unscientific' subjectivism that would be possibly questioned by philosophy, this behavioural pattern classification system and a focus on the 'organicist' body of medical sciences, the field of psy "forbids philosophy from furnishing the answer, [to] the question 'What is psychology?' [Which] becomes 'In doing what they do, what do psychologists hope to accomplish?'" (Canguilhem, 2016, p. 212). According to Guéry and Deleule (2014), *psy*-discourses are not just an ideological reflection of a capitalist mode of production. Rather, they become an indispensable gear in the social machinery that moves such ideological mechanisms. Ideology and *pathos*, in psychopathology, are deeply intertwined, with its foundations evident both in the subject assumed as normal and the subject assumed as ill, as well as in the aims of the therapeutic treatment (Federici, 2020).

Whilst the 'cure' and 'ease of suffering' may be the core aim of much, if not all, clinical practice, and the fact that such a foundation to the clinic can be at times an indisputable debate, the very understanding of what is suffering and why it needs to be 'eliminated' or even 'cured' carries with itself a heavy ideological charge. To this, Canguilhem offers an ironic yet relevant comment: "It is rather vulgarly, then, that philosophy poses to psychology the question: tell me what you aim for so that I may find out what you are?" (Canguilhem, 2016, p. 212). Here, then, the contextual debate over what is suffering and how it accompanies the discourses of normality and pathology is also a point in which psychoanalysis offers its unique approach through the psychoanalytical understanding of the symptom—not isolated, not universal, but particular and yet, in relation to a wider social, political and discursive context.

Beyond a Cartesian dualism, and far from being monistic, Freudian and Lacanian psychoanalysis then offers to the field of psy the innovation of speech and the performative aspect of the narration of one's own experience, as well as an understanding of the symptom as relating to demands of recognition that are always produced through the social bond. The early term of 'deferred action' (*Nachträglichkeit*) introduced by Freud in the 'Project for a Scientific Psychology', in 1895, when discussing the case of Emma, already brings attention to the weight of the narrative and speech over psychic reality, stressing how history, and poignantly one's own history, can be constructed retroactively. Such a movement marks a crucial component of the psychoanalytic view of subjective formation, much evidenced in the Lacanian use of the term '*parlêtre*', the speaking-being, in which the lived experience is harnessed on a body that speaks, this being the condition for subjectivity. Birman (2003) speaks of three core 'de-centrings' brought in by psychoanalysis to the world of thought and, specifically, to philosophy. I find Birman's reading useful when thinking, psychosocially, 'why psychoanalysis?', and will move into incorporating his views into our argument that follows.

Since Freud, it is in the unconscious—or in what lies beyond a conscious *Ich*—that psychoanalysis is anchored. The unconscious is, for Freud (1923), the first 'shibboleth' of psychoanalysis, "the fundamental premise of psycho-analysis; and it alone makes it possible for psycho-analysis to understand the pathological processes in mental life" (Freud, 1923, p. 13). The unconscious, as Freud suggests as early as 1894, repeating it in 1915, 1920 and explicating in 1923, "does not coincide with the repressed" (Freud, 1923, p. 18). Rather, "it is still true that all that is repressed is *Ucs.*, but not all that is *Ucs.* is repressed" (Freud, 1923, p. 18). There is, as Freud repetitively reminds us, a part of the ego that is unconscious and not related to repression or meaning; it is an 'I' beyond itself. A clinic that operates with a subject of the unconscious is, therefore, a clinic that works through the repetitions and pains, as well as the possibilities on the horizon, of such an 'I' beyond itself. In other words, psychoanalysis is, or can be, as I will move into arguing, a creative practice between 'beings' and 'becomings'.

The more general contributions of psychoanalysis to both philosophy and the sciences of the 'psy' (psychiatry, psychologies as well as neurology and neurosciences) are, according to Birman (2003), fundamentally: (1) *the unconscious activity* and (2) *the manifestations of such activity*. Within these novel paradigms it is not solely a 'divided subject' that emerges, which earlier philosophical texts were already proposing in their different approaches; for example from the Cartesian to the Kantian subjects, human 'wholeness' had been demystified in the seventeenth and eighteenth centuries. Rather, it is the production of desire (the potentialities, the complexities of symptoms and structures, etc.) in the 'being in the world' of an individual that is then understood through a systematic mapping of the psychic and subjective dynamics. In 'An Outline of Psychoanalysis', written in 1938, Freud starts off addressing this very point at which his psychoanalytic works were arriving. Freud writes:

> Psychoanalysis makes a basic assumption, the discussion of which is reserved to philosophical thought but the justification for which lies in its results. We know two kinds of things about what we call our psyche (or mental life): firstly, its bodily organ and scene of action, the brain (or nervous system) and, on the other hand, our acts of consciousness, which are immediate data and cannot be further explained by any sort of description. Everything that lies between is unknown to us, and the data do not include any direct relation between these two terminal points of our knowledge. If it existed, it would at the most afford an exact localization of the processes of consciousness and would give us no help towards understanding them. (Freud, 1938, pp. 144–145)

Here Freud acknowledges the idea of consciousness assumed by his work and that it also runs along the side of, if not against, a scientific tradition that tends—as it already did in the late 1800s—to localise acts of consciousness in the brain and, at that time, in the nervous system. Psychoanalysis brings to light the psychic apparatus and, with it, is able to raise questions that are particular to knowledge after psychoanalysis, different to other forms of divided subject or of subjectivity as carved through the social bond that could be proposed without this psychoanalytic 'mapping'.[2] Freud was not a philosopher, "but he ended up by constructing psychoanalysis as a new field of knowledge, which formulated new presuppositions in regards to subjectivity. His thought is directly linked to philosophical thought through the problems psychoanalysis posed to philosophy" (Birman, 2003, p. 16). In 'Lecture XXXV The Question of a *Weltanschauung*', part of the *New Introductory Lectures*,

[2] For example, in the fields of social and political sciences, the phenomenon of racism can be unpacked through psychoanalytic lenses; whilst in the clinical setting psychoanalysis would find unconscious marks of symptoms that have brought the patient into any particular care setting or analytic space. Fanon (1952) and the Brazilian black feminist Lélia Gonzáles (1984), for example, were pioneer scholars of the unconscious reverberations of racism and coloniality in the Freud-Lacan tradition.

Freud (1933a) opposes psychoanalysis to philosophy. Psychoanalysis, unlike philosophy, was not for Freud a *Weltanschauung*, the German term to which Freud offers a careful simple explanation as "an intellectual construction which solves all the problems of our existence uniformly on the basis of one overriding hypothesis, which, accordingly, leaves no question unanswered and in which everything that interests us finds its fixed place" (Freud, 1933b, p. 158). Freud points out that this 'view of the universe' was not the intention of psychoanalysis, since just by being a branch of psychology, psychoanalysis was, rather, more justifiably to be subjected to the 'scientific' *Weltanschauung*; yet, this 'scientific' view of the world was not really appropriate to the psychoanalytic cause. And that is "due to the procedures present in the scientific discourse, psychoanalysis would turn itself over the research of circumscribed objects, whilst philosophy had endeavoured always towards the totality of the being and of the real" (Birman, 2003, p. 9). Such a conception of philosophy is naturally debatable, but it marks one of Freud's later understandings of the status of the psychoanalytic discourse as something 'else'. Psychoanalysis is not a philosophy, nor can it be 'only' a psychology.

Upon this last point, the extract of Freud's 'An Outline of Psychoanalysis' quoted above reveals a conversation with the scientific status of psychoanalytic work. Freud is clear when arguing that even if more advanced scientific work enabled the localisation of consciousness 'inside' the brain, the experience of consciousness and of the unconscious would not change. And along with this, the 'point' or the 'justification' of psychoanalysis also does not change. And that would be because psychoanalysis, differently to neurosciences, 'deals with something else': psychoanalysis is not trying to produce a theory of the world and life and it also should not be bound to the medical-scientific discourse. That is, as mentioned previously, it may be the narrative offered to experience and the performative aspect of subjectivity that matter in the analytic experience, more than any 'verifiable' or 'arguable' reality.

Even when not particularly endeavouring to trace a whole new system of meanings, truths or theories about the universe or anything in it, Freudian psychoanalysis still was capable, under its due limitations of being first and foremost a clinical practice, of shaking if not shifting certain paradigms around the conception of a self (Ricoeur, 2008). With the psychoanalytic unconscious, a shift from the 'conscious I' to what lays beyond it and the drive become the regulators of psychic experience. Birman lists the three different meanings of the paradigmatic de-centrings inaugurated by Freud as: "1) from consciousness to the unconscious; 2) from the 'I' to the other; 3) from consciousness, the 'I' and the unconscious to the drive" (Birman, 2003, p. 60). What psychoanalysis adds to theory and to the clinic and where it diverges from other mainstream clinical practices is precisely an account of the psyche-soma that puts consciousness and individualism in question. To this list, following the 'vibrational moments' we will track down across Freud and Lacan's theories of anxiety and a Guattarian-feminist critique of psychoanalysis via Lygia Clark, I add: 4) from the Other to the vibrational, affective 'full-void' Real. Let's keep that in our pockets.

## From an Abyss-within to a Horizon-beyond

When concluding the video interview *Une Politique de la Folie*, from 1989, Tosquelles—the Catalan anarcho-syndicalist psychiatrist who founded Institutional Psychotherapy in France—leaves us with a 'prophetisation': that the proletariat should remain connected to the unconscious, rather than aim at gaining consciousness [*rester branché sur l'inconscient et non sur la prise de conscience*] *en route* to emancipation. Freud, Tosquelles (1991) argues, initially thought that the subject could become conscious of their unconscious and unknown problems, formulating a truth that would relieve suffering. Yet, Freud himself, Tosquelles suggests, changed his mind by the 1930s, disenchanted with the focus on gaining consciousness in favour of gaining unconsciousness. It is no secret that his was a Lacanian flavoured Freud, or a 'French Freud' (Turkle, 1998).[3] *Is the psychoanalytic unconscious, however, an abyss-within the subject or a horizon-beyond oneself?*

[3]Tosquelles was a colleague and mentor of Jean Oury at the hospital in Saint-Alban. Oury later was in charge of the La Borde clinic, where Guattari worked and learned. Tosquelles and Oury are major influences in the praxis of 'schizoanalysis', which is a twist Guattari proposed along with Deleuze of psychoanalysis, institutional psychotherapy and radical politics. Tosquelles and Jean Oury used to distribute copies of Lacan's doctoral thesis in psychiatry at the clinic in Saint Alban. They also quizzed new practitioners on their knowledge of the French psychoanalyst's work (Dosse, 2010).

In Freud's 1933 *New Introductory Lectures*, Lecture XXXI 'The Dissection of the Psychical Personality', we find a final version of the famous line and psychoanalytic motto he first presented in *The Ego and the Id*, in 1923: *Wo Es War, Soll Ich Werden*. "Where Id was, there ego shall be", in the original English translation by James Strachey. What Freud was proposing was that psychoanalysis' "intention is, indeed, to strengthen the ego, to make it more independent of the super-ego, to widen its field of perception and enlarge its organization, so that it can appropriate fresh portions of the id" (Freud, 1933a, p. 80). Whilst this very passage can attest to the psychoanalytic contract with a certain kind of subjective adaptation—one that would allow a liberation of oneself from an imposing super-ego in the production of a more autonomous, 'strong' ego, generating an individual of liberties, less repressions and perhaps very suitable for the demands of a global neoliberal capitalist society—it can equally attest to the contrary of adaptation to internalised morality. This very passage also reads as a definition of the psychoanalytic project and clinic as an expansion, a modification of the sense of self, making it less stiff and nailed onto the Law, capable of entering an ethical relationship to what extends beyond one's consciousness.

In the nuance of the ambiguity of this passage rests my bet with psychoanalysis. What does psychoanalysis do, or what can it do, that addresses the battles of psychic and psychosomatic suffering and, at the same time, decentres the modern humanist subject, opening possibilities for the creation of new ways of living, of new worlds? Can the psychoanalytic clinic of anxiety, thus, move from the level of an alienating subjective 'estrangement' to an 'entanglement'? It is in this midst that I anchor a question: *What can anxiety do?*

Anxiety, to Freud, *Angst*, was different to fear (*Furcht*) for it had no object. It is a suffering, a discontent, an affect without a clear reason or focus that mobilises both psyche and soma. *Angst*, in Strachey's translation of Freud into English, becomes 'anxiety' and not 'anguish', a move he justifies both in terms of the medical history of the term anxiety and of its Latin root evoking choking, making of anxiety a powerfully descriptive word for the sensation of this affect. He writes:

> There is, however, a well-established psychiatric, or at least medical, use of the English 'anxiety', going back (so the *Oxford Dictionary* tells us) to the middle of the seventeenth century. Indeed, the psychiatric use of the two words brings to light their parallel origins. '*Angst*' is akin to '*eng*', the German word for 'narrow', 'restricted'; 'anxiety' is derived from the Latin '*angere*', 'to throttle' or 'squeeze'; in both cases the reference is to the choking feelings which characterize severe forms of the psychological state in question. A still more acute condition is described in English by the word 'anguish', which has the same derivation; and it is to be remarked that Freud in his French papers uses the kindred word '*angoisse*' (as well as the synonymous '*anxiété*') to render the German '*Angst*'. (Strachey, 1962, pp. 116–117)

The word '*angoisse*' rather than *anxiété* (the word utilised by Lacan, in which Freud's translations first appeared in French) could also be more accurately translated as 'anguish' in English. In other Latin-rooted languages, such as Spanish, Portuguese and Italian, the choice in translation of both Freud and Lacan matches 'anguish' more closely in the words *angústia* and *angoscia*. Yet, the translation of Lacan's seminars into English also works with 'anxiety' and this is my choice in this cartographic effort, echoing Strachey's remarks about the medical history of 'anxiety' and the potency of a 'grammar' of psychic suffering. As it navigates translations and a telling medicalised history that marks its psychoanalytic journey, anxiety is a central theme in psychoanalytic literature and one I am venturing into in search of the creative potencies of psychoanalysis.

Lacan, in 1957, at the height of his structuralism, interprets Freud's aphorism—*Wo Es War, Soll Ich Werden*—with a slight twist, one he believed to be of a more truly Freudian inclination than that of the then dominating Ego Psychologists, Melanie Klein, and, in a broad sense, British analysts—those he accused of 'Freudery' [*fofreudisme*]. Instead of focusing on strengthening the ego, his version, as he writes in 'The Instance of the Letter in the Unconscious, or Reason Since Freud' is: "Where it was, I must come into being" (Lacan, 1957 [2006], p. 435). Lacan sees the Freudian discovery as a lesson that tells us we cannot ignore the 'radical eccentricity' of the self within itself. Not too long after, in his Seminar VII, *The Ethics of Psychoanalysis*, delivered between 1959 and 1960, Lacan discusses this aphorism once again, now to posit the ethics of psychoanalysis as beyond the morality of the super-ego, or of the morality of the Symbolic, and instead, involving an encounter with one's desire. In his words: "That 'I' which is supposed to come to be where 'it' was, and which analysis has taught us to evaluate, is nothing more than that whose root we already found in the 'I' which asks itself what it wants" (Lacan, 1959–1960 [1997], p. 7). The kind of ethics psychoanalysis mobilised in its clinical course was, to Lacan, an ethics of the Real. The Freudian contribution to the field of ethics, thus, is this encounter and a positioning of the subject vis-à-vis the Real; in Lacan's words:

> More than once at the time when I was discussing the symbolic and the imaginary and their reciprocal interaction, some of you wondered what after all was "the real." Well, as odd as it may seem to that superficial opinion which assumes any inquiry into ethics must concern the field of the ideal, if not of the unreal, I, on the contrary, will proceed instead from the other direction by going more deeply into the notion of the real. Insofar as Freud's position constitutes progress here, the question of ethics is to be articulated from the point of view of the location of man in relation to the real. (Lacan, 1959–1960 [1997], p. 11)

Anxiety, as Lacan teaches in his Seminar X *Anxiety*, delivered between 1962 and 1963, is precisely an affect that sits between desire and *jouissance* (Lacan, 1962–1963 [2016], p. 175); it is an encounter with the Real that mobilises or squeezes the subject between a Symbolically wrapped delineation of oneself, which hangs by a thread once the Imaginary fantasy of consistency fails, and the vastness and abyss that extend beyond oneself, the Real. Interestingly, it is anxiety precisely that is shunted out of diagnostic manuals and statistics when the biological and pharmaceutical paradigms of psychiatry gain strength over psychoanalysis after the late-1970s with the publication of the DSM-III (Diagnostic and Statistical Manual of Mental Disorders) in the United States. This encounter with the Real is then mediated by an ideological grammar, inaugurating a politics of affect that resonates on the possibilities of an ethical standing in relation to this abyss beyond oneself. The experience of anxiety, so central to the psychoanalytic course, is pathologised and locked into a state of estrangement, without, however, opening up to possible new ways of living. This, as we can observe in this cartographic exercise, reveals a type of alienation, an affective alienation Deleuze (1992) calls a 'dividualisation'. Perhaps Tosquelles would see it as a state where you gain neither consciousness nor unconsciousness; rather, one that is bound to a modulating external grammar, without roots, branches and leaves—let alone an ever-changing rhizome for an unconscious.

When Lacan, in 1957, characterises the unconscious as the Other's discourse (Lacan, 1957 [2006], p. 436), subjectivity is explicitly oriented in relation to an Other that is equated to the Law, to language and to a radical alterity. The Other is an 'other' not limited to identification or a projection of the level of the ego, but a wider presence carved into the Symbolic realm towards which a dialectical relation leaves a gap for the subject to come into being. If the unconscious is the Other's discourse, the Real is subsumed within its limits and 'being' leaves not much room for novel 'becomings'. If the Real is a real of 'being' and not of 'becoming', then it reveals a subtle and yet still alienating disconnection. This is what Guattari found troublesome in Lacanian structuralist psychoanalysis and wished to take further in his clinical practice and conceptual work. This transposition echoes my critique of the process of subjectivation, relationality, sociability and overall bio-politics anchored in a modern humanist and patriarchal framework found in the roots of psychoanalysis, in which a struggle for recognition by the Other modulates and locks all possibilities of being within its orbit.

Guattari learns from Lacan that desire is not 'individual' and that subjectivity is not individual either (Sauvagnargues, 2016). Whilst Lacan's 'transidividual' unconscious from the early Rome Discourse (Lacan, 1953) presents us with a notion of desire that goes beyond the relational Imaginary-to-Imaginary/ ego-to-ego field of possibilities—or really opening to a world beyond identification so clearly in his critiques of Ego-Psychology, for example—we still find an unconscious trapped into the universalism of 'lack' that derives from his structuralist interpretation of

Freud. Rosi Braidotti, across her many publications and teachings (see Braidotti, 2011), composes an argument for a 'nomadic subject'—one project that reflects the demands of post/decolonial and eco-feminist ethics, not reliant on human exceptionalism and the universalist 'Same' of modern humanism, nor on lack and castration—which is constructed from her alignment, as a feminist scholar, to Deleuze and Guattari's 'becomings', or *devenir*. The Guattarian engagement with psychoanalysis, alive in his clinical practice, moves beyond Lacan as it does not trust in the theoretical domination of the universal signifier, not reducing "the signifying assemblage as a symbolic order and [assuming] the place of the father as a master signifier, the Other that found the symbolic order" (Sauvagnargues, 2016, p. 144). Guattari shows us that this reliance on the master signifier of the father is not neutral, but a mechanism of production of a certain modulation of desire: this mode of production, reproduction, extraction and separation dubbed by the Brazilian psychoanalyst Suely Rolnik (2017) as 'the pimping of Life'. Following such critique, or holding onto this ethical disposition, we find that the orbit of the Other and its embedded universalisms does not suffice as a ground in which to account for the Real, for ruptures, affects and excesses; once such orbit does not suffice for any more radical decolonial or eco-feminist emancipatory psycho-politics beyond the 'pimping of Life' (Rolnik, 2015, 2017, 2019; Preciado, 2018).

In this sense, 'gaining unconsciousness' or encountering the Real that appears in anxiety entails opening up to common 'becomings', reorienting the clinic towards the production of a *co-poietic sinthôme*.[4] In doing so, I diverge from the (feminist and queer-informed) suggestion of the Argentinean psychoanalyst Patricia Gherovici (2018), who, in her critique of hegemonic treatment methods such as CBT (Cognitive-Behavioural Therapy), proposes further 'castration' as an analytic solution to anxiety. Instead of just renouncing the possibility of 'having it' within a phallic episteme of sexual difference, I set out to map possibilities that

[4] *Sinthôme* is a neologism rewriting the symptom, which Lacan introduces in Seminar XXIII. It consists of a creative solution in the montage of the excesses of *jouissance* beyond the logic of Oedipal castration. As such, it does not call for the clinical technique of interpretation, as it rests outside the structural diagnosis, calling for a singular clinical engagement via constructions and punctuations, or the 'cut' in the session.

veer away from the Oedipal order altogether. In this axis—Oedipus, affective alienation and interpretation—I look for an alternative route to the status of 'rupture' in the psychoanalytic clinic. Moving, thus, from a clinic of the estranged 'dividual' to an entangled, situated subject. As such, by embracing 'vibration' I move away from Oedipal configurations in this proposition of a creative clinic of anxiety; and, although this book is not mainly focused on questions of feminism in and out of psychoanalysis, I hope this clinical and conceptual discussion is fruitful to feminist figurations of all kinds.

## References

Berrios, G. E. (1996). *The History of Mental Symptoms: Descriptive Psychopathology Since the Nineteenth Century*. Cambridge University Press.

Birman, J. (2003). *Freud e a Filosofia*. Zahar.

Braidotti, R. (2011). *Nomadic Theory. The Portable Rosi Braidotti*. Columbia University Press.

Canguilhem, G. (1991). *The Normal and the Pathological*. Zone Books.

Canguilhem, G. (2016). What Is Psychology. *Foucault Studies, 21*, 200–213.

Deleuze, G. (1992). Postscript on Societies of Control. *October, 59*, 3–7.

Dosse, F. (2010). *Gilles Deleuze & Félix Guattari: Intersecting Lives*. Columbia University Press.

Fanon, F. (1952). *Peau noire, masques blancs*. Éditions du Seuil.

Federici, S. (2020). *Beyond the Periphery of the Skin: Rethinking, Remaking, and Reclaiming the Body in Contemporary Capitalism*. PM Press/Kairos.

Foucault, M. (2008). *Mental Illness and Psychology*. University of California Press.

Freud, S. (1894, June 6). Draft E. How Anxiety Originates. In *The Complete Letters of Sigmund Freud to Wilhelm Fliess, 1887–1904* (pp. 78–83).

Freud, S. (1895). A Reply to Criticisms of My Paper on Anxiety Neurosis. In *The Standard Edition of the Complete Psychological Works of Sigmund Freud, Volume III (1893–1899): Early Psycho-Analytic Publications* (pp. 119–139).

Freud, S. (1915). The Unconscious. In *The Standard Edition of the Complete Psychological Works of Sigmund Freud, Volume XIV (1914–1916): On the History of the Psycho-Analytic Movement, Papers on Metapsychology and Other Works* (pp. 159–215).

Freud, S. (1917). Introductory Lectures on Psycho-Analysis. In *The Standard Edition of the Complete Psychological Works of Sigmund Freud, Volume XVI (1916–1917): Introductory Lectures on Psycho-Analysis (Part III)* (pp. 241–463).

Freud, S. (1920). Beyond the Pleasure Principle. In *The Standard Edition of the Complete Psychological Works of Sigmund Freud, Volume XVIII (1920–1922): Beyond the Pleasure Principle, Group Psychology and Other Works* (pp. 1–64).

Freud, S. (1923). The Ego and the Id. In *The Standard Edition of the Complete Psychological Works of Sigmund Freud, Volume XIX (1923–1925): The Ego and the Id and Other Works* (pp. 1–66).

Freud, S. (1933a). Lecture XXXI The Dissection of the Psychical Personality. New Introductory Lectures on Psycho-Analysis. In *The Standard Edition of the Complete Psychological Works of Sigmund Freud, Volume XXII (1932–1936): New Introductory Lectures on Psycho-Analysis and Other Works* (pp. 1–182).

Freud, S. (1933b). Lecture XXXV The Question of a Weltanschauung. New Introductory Lectures on Psycho-Analysis. In *The Standard Edition of the Complete Psychological Works of Sigmund Freud, Volume XXII (1932–1936): New Introductory Lectures on Psycho-Analysis and Other Works* (pp. 1–182).

Freud, S. (1938). An Outline of Psycho-Analysis. In *The Standard Edition of the Complete Psychological Works of Sigmund Freud, Volume XXIII (1937–1939): Moses and Monotheism, An Outline of Psycho-Analysis and Other Works* (pp. 139–208).

Gallagher, C. (1996). High Anxiety – A Theoretical and Clinical Challenge to Psychoanalysis. *The Letter, 6*(Spring), 1–23.

Gherovici, P. (2018). Anxious? Castration Is the Solution! *Psychoanalytic Inquiry, 38*(1), 83–90.

Gonzáles, L. (1984). *Racismo e Sexismo na Cultura Brasileira* (pp. 223–244). Revista Ciências Sociais Hoje, Anpocs.

Guéry, F., & Deleule, D. (2014). *The Productive Body*. Zero Books.

Klein, M. ([1948] 1988). The Theory of Anxiety and Guilt. In M. Klein (Ed.), *Envy and Gratitude and Other Works 1946–1963*. Virago Press.

Lacan, J. (1953). The Function and Field of Speech and Language in Psychoanalysis. In *Écrits:* The First 'Complete Edition in English (2006) [Trans. B. Fink]. W.W. Norton and Company.

Lacan, J. (1957). The Instance of the Letter in the Unconscious, or Reason Since Freud. In *Écrits:* The First Complete Edition in English (2006) [Trans. B. Fink]. W.W. Norton and Company.

Lacan, J. (1960). The Subversion of the Subject and the Dialectic of Desire in the Freudian Unconscious. In *Écrits:* The First Complete Edition in English (2006) [Trans. B. Fink]. W.W. Norton and Company.

Lacan, J. (1997). *The Seminar of Jacques Lacan. Book VII: The Ethics of Psychoanalysis. 1959–1960*. W.W. Norton & Company.

Lacan, J. (2016). *Anxiety. The Seminar of Jacques Lacan Book X* (J.-A. Miller, Ed.). Polity Press.

Marcuse, H. (1969). *Eros & Civilization*. Sphere Books.

Middleton, H., & Moncrieff, J. (2019). Critical Psychiatry: A Brief Overview. *BJPsych Advances, 25*(1), 47–54.

Preciado, P. B. ([2018] 2019). La isquierda bajo la piel. Um prólogo para Suely Rolnik. In S. Rolnik (Ed.), *Esferas da Insurreição: notas para uma vida não cafetinada*. n-1.

Proctor, G. (2008). CBT: The Obscuring of Power in the Name of Science. *European Journal of Psychotherapy and Counselling, 10*(3), 231–245.

Ricoeur, P. (2008). *Freud and Philosophy: An Essay on Interpretation*. Yale University Press.

Robcis, C. (2021). *Disalienation: Politics, Philosophy, and Radical Psychiatry in Postwar France*. University of Chicago Press.

Rolnik, S. (2015). Beyond the Colonial Unconscious. *Art and Education* [Online]. https://www.artandeducation.net/classroom/video/66076/suely-rolnik-beyond-colonial-unconscious

Rolnik, S. (2017, November). The Spheres of Insurrection: Suggestions for Combating the Pimping of Life. *E-flux* [Online]. https://www.e--flux.com/journal/86/163107/the-spheres-of-insurrection-suggestions-for-combating-the-pimping-of-life/

Rolnik, S. (2019). *Esferas da Insurreição: notas para uma vida não cafetinada*. n-1.

Rose, N. (2018). *Our Psychiatric Future: The Politics of Mental Health*. Polity Press.

Rustin, M. (2015). Why Klein-Lacan Dialogue Is Difficult. In J. Borossa, C. Bronstein, & C. Pajaczkowska (Eds.), *The New Klein-Lacan Dialogues*. Karnac.

Sauvagnargues, A. (2016). *Artmachines: Deleuze, Guattari, Simondon*. Edinburgh University Press.

Shorter, E. (2005). *A Historical Dictionary of Psychiatry*. Oxford University Press.

Soler, C. (2014). *Lacanian Affects: The Function of Affect in Lacan's Work*. Routledge.

Strachey, J. (1962). The Term 'Angst' and Its English Translation. In *The Standard Edition of the Complete Psychological Works of Sigmund Freud, Volume III (1893–1899): Early Psycho-Analytic Publications* (pp. 116–117).

Tosquelles, F. (1991). Une politique de la folie. *Chimères. Revue des schizoanalyses, 13*(Automne), 66–81.

Turkle, S. (1998). *Psychoanalytic Politics: Freud's French Revolution*. Basic Books.

# 5

# Libidinal Excesses

In the first pages of 'An Autobiographic study', from 1925, Freud narrates his collaborative work with Breuer, hinting at a divisive trait between the two doctors' personalities when writing: "The theory which we had attempted to construct in the *Studies* remained, as I have said, very incomplete; and in particular we had scarcely touched on the problem of aetiology, on the question of the ground in which the pathogenic process takes root" (Freud, 1925, p. 23). The ground, the basis, the context. Freud was concerned with what allowed for psychic processes to take place, and this was a matter dealt with in a number of his texts, when both internal and external realities were negotiated in manners that would permit certain traits, actions and, ultimately, symptoms to emerge. Psychoanalysis speaks of a subject harnessed to the world and in its theories and practices, psychic structure and the lived experience carry the same weight.

Anxiety, which is not a symptom, but an affect, is mostly acknowledged through its appearance on the body, confusing any delineated spaces of the symptom, affect, internal and external worlds, psyche and soma. This affective riddle is studied in detail in what follows. In this chapter, I offer close critical readings of Freud's key theoretical formulations of anxiety, which are revealed in a contrast with mainstream



A. C. Minozzo, *Anxiety as Vibration*, Studies in the Psychosocial,
https://doi.org/10.1007/978-3-031-62856-6_5

psychiatric nosology. I work with less popular nineteenth century texts and letters known as 'pre-psychoanalytic' works, all the way through to Freud's 1930s final remarks on the topic of anxiety. Through the method of close readings, it is possible to grasp the nuanced transformations of Freud's theories of the 'grounds' of anxiety across four decades, in the build-up to a formulation of anxiety as vibration—or anxiety as an affect of rupture that vibrates through the subject and beyond oneself, an affect of entanglement. The pieces selected operate as an archive, offering insight into the 'grounds' of anxiety; their importance is given by how 'anxiety' is the kernel of the psychoneuroses in Freudian psychoanalysis. The following close readings of Freud will enable us to rescue specific 'vibrational moments' in his theories of anxiety, in which an anxiety that is not relying on Oedipus is more apparent both at the very beginning of his writings and at the very end, as follows.

## Freud's Works on Anxiety

Already in Freud's letters to Wilhelm Fliess, an attempt to unravel the complexities of anxiety (*angst*, in the German original) was being traced. The mechanisms of this affect and its connections to a discharge of libido, repression and fear followed Freud's works over decades, from the end of the nineteenth century to his last years of his life in the early 1930s, marking different stages of the development of his theories on anxiety, which emerges as a direct neurotic repression and moves towards a more refined understanding of the importance and variations of this puzzling affect. In the seminal 'Inhibitions, Symptoms and Anxiety', 1926, Freud's delineation of the aetiology and symptomatology of anxiety presents the first important shift in this understanding, as his clinical experience was then able to suggest that "it was anxiety which produced repression and not, as I formerly believed, repression which produced anxiety" (Freud, 1926, pp. 108–109). Anxiety, at a point that succeeded his works on the libidinal economy surrounding the life and death drives in 'Beyond the Pleasure Principle' (1920), was seen as a form of psychic protection against threats to one's integrity. It is precisely over the variations of such threats, their origin and their relation to the manifestation of a subsequent anxiety that Freud mapped concepts such as realistic anxiety, neurotic anxiety, moral anxiety, primary anxiety, castration anxiety and signal anxiety. As this chapter will demonstrate, it is only in the mid-1920s that the Oedipal metaphor marks the Freudian theory of anxiety in relation to castration and, consequently, sexual difference. Anxiety seemingly wears many hats in the Freudian oeuvre, all of them as an 'excess'—either in the form of an abyss within or of a vast horizon beyond the limits of the 'I' (the *Ich*, ego). In what follows, I stay as close as possible to Freud, grasping his rationale and logic according to his own words, moving into a clear understanding of Lacan's contributions to the topic in the next chapter—and, subsequently, a debate on the limits of psychoanalytic theory to contemporary praxis.

## Letters to Fliess and Late Nineteenth Century

Two letters, known as drafts A and B, pose important points in Freud's early theories on anxiety, specifically anxiety neurosis. In draft A1, from 1892, a text in bullet points, sexuality and repression already form his hypothesis. In draft B, from the same year, 1892, Freud was working on an actiology of neuroses, and *chronic state* and an *attack of anxiety* are mentioned as two different manifestations of anxiety that can be combined in symptoms that revolve around the body (i.e. hypochondria, agoraphobia, etc.) and the *sexual noxa* (Freud, 1892, p. 183). According to Freud, the latter means events or circumstances that disrupt some sort of 'natural' flow of sexual satisfaction. It is, however, only a couple of years later that Freud elaborated in more detail his work in progress on the equation of neurosis, sexuality, repression and anxiety. In an 1894 short letter to Fliess, known as Draft E, Freud takes his friend through his thinking process. There he explores anxiety neurosis, which he at first and for the next coming decades understands as linked with sexuality. Sexuality, as it will unfold across his work, starts off as a bodily excess he names 'libido' and moves, later, into a modification of the idea of 'castration' in relation to the 'phallus', where anxiety is placed.

Freud writes: "All I know about it is this: It quickly became clear to me that the anxiety of my neurotic patients had a great deal to do with sexuality; and in particular it struck me with what certainty *coitus interruptus* practiced on a woman leads to anxiety neurosis" (Freud, 1894a, p. 78). *Coitus interruptus*, which was a common practice at the time, over half a century before the popularisation of the contraceptive pill, caused particular anxiety, both in men and women (following the heteronormative view of sexuality displayed in these letters). However, this first observation soon after called for revision, since anxiety would appear even in people not worrying about pregnancy. Another factor emerges in Freud's early observations that will carry a certain weight in his theories of anxiety, that of its connections with the physical body, at this point solely linked with sexual satisfaction. Freud spells out the following:

> [...] anxiety neurosis affects women who are anaesthetic in coitus just as much as sensitive ones. This is most peculiar, but it can only mean that the source of the anxiety is not to be looked for in the psychic sphere. It must accordingly lie in the physical sphere: it is a physical factor in sexual life that produces anxiety. (Freud, 1894a, p. 78)

Freud reports having followed a variety of cases in which sexuality and anxiety would be connected, ranging from a 'virginal anxiety' until the "anxiety of men *who go beyond their desire or strength*, older people whose potency is diminishing, but who nevertheless forcibly bring about coitus" (Freud, 1894a, p. 79). However, he does not provide any detail of such cases. Yet, such wide range of cases were, to him, connected by "an accumulation of physical sexual tension" (Freud, 1894a, p. 79) that lead to anxiety via a 'detour' of such accumulation and its discharge, in which this accumulated tension is 'transformed' into anxiety. There is, thus, right from the start of his understanding a path forming through a physical excess that is left unsatisfied firstly physically, but for reasons that could be physical or not, and then accumulated and psychically transformed into something else; this something else would be the manifestation of anxiety symptoms. Anxiety and the drive are early partners in psychoanalytic thinking.

The physicality of anxiety was stressed in this very early text and as Freud was developing his work on melancholia at the time of writing this letter, he offered an interesting parallel between these two states, which are demarcated precisely by the duality of psychic and physical.

> Quite particularly often, melancholies have been anaesthetic. They have no desire for coitus (and no sensation in connection with it), but they have a great longing for love in its psychic form—one might say, psychic erotic tension; where this accumulates and remains unsatisfied, melancholia develops. This, then, would be the counterpart to anxiety neurosis. Where physical sexual tension accumulates—anxiety neurosis. Where psychic sexual tension accumulates—melancholia. (Freud, 1894a, p. 80)

Melancholia, here, is enticed by an external presence that results in an internal response being quantitatively re-balanced, since "for that purpose any reaction suffices that diminishes the inner psychic excitation by the same quantum" (Freud, 1894a, p. 80). Anxiety, on the other hand, derives from an internal source of tension that lies in the body—sexual drive, hunger, thirst—and the difference here being that only very 'specific' things could quench and satisfy these needs, preventing their occurrence again in 'the organs concerned' to each need. By tracing this path, Freud provided an interesting theory of psyche-soma. Connecting body and psyche, a type of 'threshold' appears. Only when such threshold is reached, affective states are able to deploy psychic connections, entering, as he puts it, "into relation with certain groups of ideas, which then set about producing the specific remedies" (Freud, 1894a, p. 80). The drives are the motor of psychic activity.

Sexual libido is seen as somewhat independent from the psyche at the same time as it depends upon a psychic origin. Anxiety emerges when either one's psychic reality, for example a defence mechanism that interrupts the possibility of this libido transformation "as it should be" from psyche/body to body back to psyche, or when something just physical proves to be the '*noxa*' (*coitus interruptus* as a practice, or a bodily malfunction, etc.). Anxiety arises through "the accumulation of physical tension and the prevention of discharge in the psychic direction" (Freud, 1894a, p. 82). Why anxiety, specifically, is what Freud leaves as an open question at the end of this letter, when he provides an answer that is, in a certain way, rather flimsy. Anxiety, he argues, arises, instead of anything else, as its typical symptoms resemble the very act of discharge of the accumulated sexual tension, by which he means, anxiety symptoms resemble the sexual act, so anxiety symptoms become a substituting route of discharge:

> Anxiety is the sensation of the accumulation of another endogenous stimulus, the stimulus to breathing, a stimulus incapable of being worked over psychically apart from this; anxiety might therefore be employed for accumulated physical tension in general. Furthermore, if the symptoms of anxiety neurosis are examined more closely, one finds in the neurosis disjointed pieces of a major anxiety attack: namely, mere dyspnea, mere palpitations, mere feeling of anxiety, and a combination of these. Looked at more precisely, these are the paths of innervation that the physical sexual tension ordinarily traverses even when it is about to be worked over psychically. The dyspnea and palpitations belong to coitus; and while ordinarily they are employed only as subsidiary paths of discharge, here they serve, so to speak, as the only outlets for the excitation. This is once again a kind of *conversion* in anxiety neurosis, just as occurs in hysteria (another instance of their similarity); but in hysteria it is *psychic* excitation that takes a wrong path exclusively into the somatic field, whereas here it is a *physical* tension, which cannot enter the psychic field and therefore remains on the physical path. (Freud, 1894a, p. 82)

Much of this letter gave origin to an expanded paper published that same year under the title 'On The Grounds for Detaching a Particular Syndrome From Neurasthenia Under The Description "Anxiety Neurosis"' (1894b). As the title suggests, this text is concerned mainly with setting an aetiology and mechanisms particular to neurasthenia (a popular diagnosis of the time) and what he was referring as 'anxiety neurosis', the latter being the transformed discharge of accumulated sexual tension as he had written to Fliess.

Anxiety neurosis was here being called as such "because all its components can be grouped round the chief symptom of anxiety, because each one of them has a definite relationship to anxiety" (Freud, 1894b, p. 91). The clinical symptoms identified by Freud in this paper of what would consist of an anxiety neurosis were:

1. General irritability;
2. Anxious expectation—which he saw as central to neurosis, once "we may perhaps say that here a quantum of anxiety in a freely floating state is present, which, where there is expectation, controls the choice of ideas and is always ready to link itself with any suitable ideational content" (Freud, 1894b, p. 93);
3. Anxiety attacks that are sudden and not linked to a train of ideas and a more general anxiousness, that appears as a feeling of anxiety that the patient feels as linked to a bodily function, this emerging in complaints "of 'spasms of the heart' 'difficulty in breathing' 'outbreaks of sweating' 'ravenous hunger' and such like; and, in his description, the feeling of anxiety often recedes into the background or is referred to quite unrecognizably as 'being unwell' 'feeling uncomfortable' and so on" (Freud, 1894b, p. 93);
4. Different types of anxiety attacks, for example, accompanied by breathing problems, or heart beating problems, or even ravenous hunger;
5. *pavor nocturnus* or night terrors on adults and children;
6. Vertigo;
7. Phobias related to chronic anxiousness or vertigo, ranging from physiological dangers to locomotion dangers and apparent in phobia of thunderstorms in the first case to agoraphobia in the latter, for example;
8. Digestion activities disturbances;
9. *Paraesthesias*;
10. And, finally, all the above, in either an attack or a chronic form.

Such symptoms could be easily 'confused' with that of neurasthenia, a condition popularly diagnosed after George Miller Beard, an American neurologist, described it as a problem or weakness of the actual 'nerves' (Berrios, 1996). Freud, in this paper, recognizes the potential similarities in diagnosis of cases of neurasthenia and anxiety neurosis, but he moves on to clarifying the difference between the two as resting precisely on the specific sexual origins of anxiety neurosis. What he adds in this paper, furthering from his earlier letter to Fliess, is that in many cases of anxiety neurosis, sexual desire is also lessened, adding this other layer to the 'origins' of anxiety since "the mechanism of anxiety neurosis is to be looked for in a deflection of somatic sexual excitation from the psychical sphere, and in a consequent abnormal employment of that excitation" (Freud, 1894b, p. 108). In neurasthenia, Freud signals, it can be that the 'unloading' is not as adequate (masturbation as a replacement for the 'normal coition', is the example he provides); yet, "anxiety neurosis, on the other hand, is the product of all those factors which prevent the somatic sexual excitation from being worked over psychically. The manifestations of anxiety neurosis appear when the somatic excitation which has been deflected from the psyche is expended subcortically in totally inadequate reactions" (Freud, 1894b, p. 109). By pairing, once again, the symptoms of anxiety and the physical aspects of sexual interactions (which, in this logic, must include another person, or an other), Freud "depicts the symptoms of anxiety neurosis as being in a sense surrogates of the omitted specific action following on sexual excitation" (Freud, 1894b, p. 111).

Freud will then move into differentiating, for the first time, the affect of anxiety and anxiety neurosis. Elaborating on the function of anxiety, Freud claims that the 'regular' affect of anxiety offers a certain protection against something external that cannot be dealt with accordingly. Anxiety neurosis thus is a response to an internal excess, whilst the affect of anxiety has external bearings. He writes:

> The psyche finds itself in the affect of anxiety if it feels unable to deal by appropriate reaction with a task (a danger) approaching from outside; it finds itself in the neurosis of anxiety if it notices that it is unable to even out the (sexual) excitation originating from within—that is to say, it behaves as though it were projecting that excitation outwards. The affect and its corresponding neurosis are firmly related to each other. The first is a reaction to an exogenous excitation, the second a reaction to the analogous endogenous one. The affect is a state which passes rapidly, the neurosis is a chronic one; because, while exogenous excitation operates as a constant force, in the neurosis, the nervous system is reacting against a source of excitation which is internal, whereas in the corresponding affect it is reacting against an analogous source of excitation which is external. (Freud, 1894b, p. 112)

If we make a simple parallel between what Freud proposes here and the rise in reports of anxiety by the ONS in the UK during the first COVID-19 lockdown, for instance, a less pathologised approach unfolds. The affect of anxiety is, if anything, under such Freudian lenses, a healthy reaction to overwhelming external circumstances. Such affect, rather than a 'stranger' within, qualifies an entanglement with the world, or a deep psychic, bodily, libidinal connection with it. If a complex symptomatic presentation is developed in relation to such anxiety, then the singular layers of one's drive and its bearings in the subjective positioning of the patient in the world are also involved in a complaint of high anxiety. In both cases, neurotic or not, anxiety is an affect of entanglement and depth, rather than of surface and estrangement—as qualified in the hegemonic diagnoses and treatment discourses post-1970s.

Two months after the publication of 'On The Grounds', in the January 1895 issue of the journal *Neurologisckes Zentralblatt*, Leopold Löwenfeld, a German psychiatrist, published a critique of the paper. Freud responds in the same year with the essay 'A Reply to Criticisms of My Paper on Anxiety Neurosis' (1895), picking up on his conclusions that followed from clinical observations.

> I arrived at the proposition: anxiety neurosis is created by everything which keeps somatic sexual tension away from the psychical sphere, which interferes with its being worked over psychically. If we go back to the concrete circumstances in which this factor becomes operative, we are led to assert that [sexual] abstinence, whether voluntary or involuntary, sexual intercourse with incomplete satisfaction, *coitus interruptus*, deflection of psychical interest from sexuality, and similar things, are the specific aetiological factors of the states to which I have given the name of anxiety neurosis. (Freud, 1895, p. 124)

Löwenfeld had challenged the above logic by providing cases in which anxiety neurosis emerged from singular events of fright, not sharing the sexual path suggested by Freud. Freud responds by claiming he did not doubt his colleague's cases, neither other 'official academic medicine' cases as possibilities of refusal of his hypotheses; he doubted, however, the very kind of interpretation being provided to cases by these other practitioners. So, he writes,

> if anyone wants to prove to me that in these remarks I have unduly neglected the significance of the stock aetiological factors, he must confront me with observations in which my specific factor is missing—that is, with cases in which anxiety neurosis has arisen after a psychical shock although the subject has (on the whole) led a normal *vita sexualis*. (Freud, 1895, p. 128)

Freud defends the psychoanalytic method as—it seems, at least in contrast with neuropathological methods—the only one capable of providing in depth enough interpretations that would not only prove his theory of anxiety neurosis right as really unveil symptoms once "it is impossible to pursue an aetiological investigation based on anamneses if we accept those anamneses as the patients present them, or are content with what they are willing to volunteer" (Freud, 1895, p. 129). In other words, the complaints of a surface level symptom presentation cannot be treated as the totality of this symptom. Rather, the Freudian method will trace the grounds and dynamics of symptom-formation in the unconscious.

These very early writings on anxiety, when considered together, propose two interesting entries into the notion of 'vibration' I am carving through this cartography: (1) its relation to the drive and (2) its internal and external sources of stimuli. Whilst reading Freud's almost stereotypical pairing of any symptomatology with sexuality (and an essentialist heteronormative view of such) is rather frustrating, the addition of libido, satisfaction, discharge and the overall dynamics of the drive are fundamental to his contribution to the field of psy. The subject appears as one that is marked by *jouissance*, rather than simply being a one-dimensional social subject guided by morality. When attributing to anxiety a relation to libidinal excess, Freud proposes a treatment that is fundamentally contrary to the method of symptom isolation and 'checklist' proposed by mainstream psychiatry. The subject presented here not only enjoys as they also are harnessed to the world and its contingencies and stimuli. Anxiety, as seen in these early texts, is also 'naturalised' rather than 'pathologised', appearing as a dynamic relation to the body, the unconscious and stimuli (both as a regular affect and in anxiety neurosis, as seen above). Another nuance I find interesting here is the non-reliance on sexual difference observable in these works. Elaborated before Freud delineated the Oedipus Complex, these texts do not propose different unconscious positions and symptom formation for 'men' and 'women'. Rather we are dealing with a threshold of excess that mobilises the body and psyche in anxiety. Guattari rescued these letters and Freud's 'energetic model' of the unconscious in the later years of his thinking precisely because of their non-reliance on Oedipus.

## Introductory Lectures: Lecture XXV, 1917

In the final part of his Introductory Lectures, about two decades after his initial works on anxiety neurosis, Freud provides an updated and objective account of his theory of anxiety. He sets out by proposing that whilst most people must have already experienced the 'sensation' or the 'affect' of anxiety, there is something particular in the experiences of anxiety of neurotics, and to this he will dedicate this lecture. This affect is seen by Freud as particularly complex for "there is no question that the problem of anxiety is a nodal point at which the most various and important questions converge, a riddle whose solution would be bound to throw a flood of light on our whole mental existence" (Freud, 1917, p. 393). This shared experience of anxiety both in a 'normal' and in a 'pathological' state is given more structure in this lecture, once Freud offers a distinction between 'realistic' and 'neurotic' anxieties.

Realistic anxiety, whilst being "connected with the flight reflex and [...] regarded as a manifestation of the self-preservative instinct" (Freud, 1917, p. 394), accounts for a rather rational manifestation. It makes little sense if we think that in such occasions of imminent danger, being anxious does little to help avoiding such danger, and quite the contrary, can bring about a paralysis and lack of action that could be the opposite of self-preservative. However strange this may seem, Freud points out that it is preparedness for the danger that increases one's attention and motor capacity, reading for action. Anxiety as a 'signal' is divided in two 'moments' and "the preparedness for anxiety seems [to me] to be the expedient element in what we call anxiety, and the generation of anxiety the inexpedient one" (Freud, 1917, p. 395). Our perception of these expressions of anxiety leads Freud to the central question of: What exactly is anxiety?

His answer is that anxiety is an affect. Affect, in its turn, is a complex concept that "includes in the first place particular motor innervations or discharges and secondly certain feelings; the latter are of two kinds—perceptions of the motor actions that have occurred and the direct feelings of pleasure and unpleasure which, as we say, give the affect its keynote" (Freud, 1917, p. 395). Affects, in this view, relate to the body and the psyche, touching on perception and feelings. The 'imprint' of the affect of anxiety, which is then repeated when this affect comes about, is present at the instant of birth, as well as in the 'unpleasant' separation from the mother. He writes:

> We believe that it is in the act of birth that there comes about the combination of un-pleasurable feelings, impulses of discharge and bodily sensations which has become the prototype of the effects of a mortal danger and has ever since been repeated by us as the state of anxiety. The immense increase of stimulation owing to the interruption of the renovation of the blood (internal respiration) was at the time the cause of the experience of anxiety; the first anxiety was thus a toxic one. (Freud, 1917, p. 396)

Affect, in Freudian theory, thus, has to do with an extension of oneself, mobilising perception; and a relation to the other, the mother more specifically, as a primary love and dependency object. In this discreet sense, by thinking of anxiety as an affect as such, Freud builds upon his earlier libidinal theory that accounted for stimulus that leads to anxiety as endogenous, or of an understanding of sexuality as endogenous, rather than as a 'drive'. A drive, as such, mobilises both the internal and external realms, in and out, the *extimate* (external and intimate), in Lacanian words.

The differences between the affect of anxiety, that which can be shared by anyone, and a neurotic experience of anxiety follow in this text. An 'expectant anxiety', or an anticipation of something that can happen and is undesirable, is a shared affective state in which "we find a general apprehensiveness, a kind of freely floating anxiety which is ready to attach itself to any idea that is in any way suitable, which influences judgement, selects what is to be expected, and lies in wait for any opportunity that will allow it to justify itself" (Freud, 1917, p. 398). When too much of this 'expectant anxiety' appears it "forms a regular feature of a nervous disorder to which I have given the name of 'anxiety neurosis' and which [I] include among the 'actual' neuroses" (Freud, 1917, p. 398). Freud observes that there is also another type of anxiety, phobia, that instead of being free-floating and characterised by the above-mentioned neurotic 'structure' of anxiety "is bound psychically and attached to particular objects or situations. This is the anxiety of the extremely multifarious and often very strange 'phobias'" (Freud, 1917, p. 398).

Freud's previous work on anxiety neurosis forms a base to his explanations surrounding yet another type of neurotic anxiety, that "faces us with the puzzling fact that here the connection between anxiety and a threatening danger is completely lost to view" (Freud, 1917, p. 401)—or an anxiety without 'reality' nor object. This lack of a correlation to danger leads Freud to a few hypotheses when trying to connect realist anxiety and neurotic anxiety. For example: Could there be anything the patient is in fact afraid of at the heart of their neurotic anxiety? This crucial point, later to be developed further in his 1926 text 'Inhibitions, Symptoms and Anxiety', finds its first explanation here, bringing back the previous ideas of discharge of sexual libido. Without departing from his earlier texts too drastically, Freud argues that "it is not difficult to establish the fact that expectant anxiety or general apprehensiveness is closely dependent on certain happenings in sexual life, or, let us say, certain employments of the libido" (Freud, 1917, p. 401). That would be the case in the most varied contexts, even when sexuality is bound to 'cultural differences'; he states that "however much these relations are altered and complicated by a variety of cultural influences, it nevertheless remains true of the average of mankind that anxiety has a close connection with sexual limitation" (Freud, 1917, p. 402). All in all, these observations led him "to conclude that the deflection of the libido from its normal employment, which causes the development of anxiety, takes place in the region of somatic processes" (Freud, 1917, p. 404). What will become clearer as Freud moves along with his writing is that for him, a normal employment of libido must involve another object or an extension beyond one's own body and idea of self.

Whilst neurotic and realistic anxiety as different 'categories' proposed by Freud in this text may have different origins—the former related to 'libido put to 'abnormal' employment' and the latter 'a reaction to danger'—in the way such anxieties are felt, there is no distinction, for what is 'real' or 'dangerous' are complex categories when dealing with the unconscious. This open question is also picked up in the following decade, when Freud works with the concept of 'castration anxiety'.

It is necessary to introduce another factor that Freud presents here adding further to his theories on anxiety, that of the oppositions between the ego and libido:

> As we know, the generation of anxiety is the ego's reaction to danger and the signal for taking flight. If so, it seems plausible to suppose that in neurotic anxiety the ego is making a similar attempt at flight from the demand by its libido, that it is treating this internal danger as though it were an external one. This would therefore fulfil our expectation that where anxiety is shown there is something one is afraid of. But the analogy could be carried further. Just as the attempt at flight from an external danger is replaced by standing firm and the adoption of expedient measures of defence, so too the generation of neurotic anxiety gives place to the formation of symptoms, which results in the anxiety being bound. (Freud, 1917, p. 405)

The ego, here being confronted by some internal libidinal 'call', starts to appear as the guarantor of a certain psychic stability in the end of Freud's lecture, which ends with the debate between anxiety and repression. He asks, "what happens to the affect that was attached to the repressed idea?" (Freud, 1917, p. 403) and his answer is "that the immediate vicissitude of that affect is to be transformed into anxiety, whatever quality it may have exhibited apart from this in the normal course of events" (Freud, 1917, p. 409). Such 'discharge' into anxiety of what was repressed also follows a particular route in phobias, slightly different then in cases of other neuroses:

> In phobias, for instance, two phases of the neurotic process can be clearly distinguished. The first is concerned with repression and the changing of libido into anxiety, which is then bound to an external danger. The second consists in the erection of all the precautions and guarantees by means of which any contact can be avoided with this danger, treated as it is like an external thing. Repression corresponds to an attempt at flight by the ego from libido which is felt as a danger. A phobia may be compared to an entrenchment against an external danger which now represents the dreaded libido. (Freud, 1917, p. 410)

This 'remainder' is accounted for in Freud's most famous case of phobia, Little Hans, published in 1909 and delineating that some excess of this 'libidinal flow' not grasped by the conversion in anxiety will not be shifted onto the object even in cases of phobia. In this sense, anxiety appears to us clearly as a 'surplus' or an excess in what Freud called 'libido' that does not and cannot find total and complete grounds to be satisfied or channelled in the body (in sex, eating, drinking or other points when need and desire circle what later will be the 'drive') nor in representation, or words and symbolisation. Here we must pay special attention to the quality of this 'surplus', as it will be the grounds on which Lacan will later pin down the Real (where anxiety is located)—an excess that is not connected to desire nor satisfaction, and which is not bound by symbolisation.

In this account of anxiety, Freud is able to schematise anxiety within the topology of the 'ego' as functioning as a guarantor for subjectivity thus, gatekeeping excessive libido. This formulation is crucial to the understanding of anxiety as vibration, once it describes the psychic life of the subject formulated by psychoanalysis—one whose excesses are displaced (phobia), channelled (affect of anxiety) or accumulated (anxiety neurosis) in the body. Psyche-soma, or the subject of the drive, clearly presents a libidinal charge to ideas and representation. In this manner, and again without relying on Oedipal sexual difference, Freud challenges what is later proposed by Cognitive-Behavioural Therapy, which accounts for a non-libidinised relation to thoughts, working, instead, with an automatic body/mind model of the subject. What is also interesting in this 1917 work is that it again does away with the pathologisation of anxiety, describing so clearly that this is a fundamental affect that is formative of psychic experience. In treatment, thus, when working with a case of extreme anxiety, the ego and its function of a gatekeeper of psychic stability is the focus of the treatment. Instead of getting rid of anxiety altogether, the Freudian model implies that we work through it. This, of course, does away with the reliance on psychopharmakon as a treatment for anxiety, or a treatment for stopping the body 'feeling' anxiety.

Whilst Freud gives us a rich account of how anxiety is an integral part of psychic experience and points towards a treatment of the ego, he is yet to add his theories of the function of the Id and the superego in this equation that results in anxiety. When he does so, the Modern humanism (and patriarchal) tone of his psychoanalytic ideas becomes stronger, as I will develop next.

## Inhibitions Symptoms and Anxiety, 1926

It is in this 1926 essay that Freud outlines his most elaborate theory of anxiety, following a temporal logic that can be summarised as initially connecting anxiety as an un-discharged sexual tension; then as repressed libido. He further differentiates between anxiety being either realistic or neurotic and, finally, proposes that anxiety is a signal in the ego of a danger of disintegration. In this paper, Freud 'updates' earlier views, especially in respect to libido and anxiety, a view he now regards as "not [in] accord with the general character of anxiety as a reaction to unpleasure" (Freud, 1926, p. 161). Unpleasure, in psychoanalytic parlance, is of the order of the excessive, that which disturbs homeostasis.

The essay itself is quite contradictory and fragmented, divided in chapters and including a final addendum, where earlier concepts are summarised, reworked, rejected and confirmed, sometimes in a very circular manner. Yet, there are important points that will later be worked over by Lacan in the 1960s. Freud begins arguing about the differences between an inhibition and a symptom, which may seem simple but reveal his journey into some key dynamics of psychic structures. Parting from the common use of each term being the first of a 'non-function' and the latter a 'wrong-functioning', Freud indicates that in reality the very inhibition, or a 'non-functioning function', can be a symptom itself in the eyes of psychoanalysis. Anxiety and inhibitions are correlated. Freud explains that "some inhibitions obviously represent a relinquishment of a function because its exercise would produce anxiety" (Freud, 1926, p. 88). Whilst the inhibition to eat or towards the sexual act can take place, a symptom would be, as he offers as examples, vomiting or disgust at the idea of sex. In the clinic, mapping the function and dynamics of a symptom is a fundamental direction in the treatment. This is a way to trace the singular arrangement of one's subjectivity in relation to their psychic suffering.

For Freud, when there is a restriction of an ego-function, an inhibition takes place "the ego renounces these functions, which are within its sphere, in order not to have to undertake fresh measures of repression—in order to avoid a conflict with the id" (Freud, 1926, p. 90). Thus, we find here inhibitions being seen almost as a 'protective measure'. At the same time, inhibitions can represent self-punishment, "in order to avoid coming into conflict with the super-ego" (Freud, 1926, p. 90). Whilst inhibitions "are restrictions of the functions of the ego which have been either imposed as a measure of precaution or brought about as a result of an impoverishment of energy" (Freud, 1926, p. 90), symptoms differ by not being "a process that takes place within, or acts upon, the ego" (Freud, 1926, p. 90). Here is why Lacan will go on to say that anxiety is not a symptom, rather, it is an affect.

Freud challenges his earlier understanding of the symptom, which was by now complicated by the findings in his work on 'Beyond the Pleasure Principle' (1920):

> A symptom is a sign of, and a substitute for, an instinctual satisfaction which has remained in abeyance; it is a consequence of the process of repression. Repression proceeds from the ego when the latter—it may be at the behest of the superego—refuses to associate itself with an instinctual cathexis which has been aroused in the id. The ego is able by means of repression to keep the idea which is the vehicle of the reprehensible impulse from becoming conscious. (Freud, 1926, p. 91)

This view of the symptom in relation to unpleasure as what is actually being 'looked for' instinctually posits that a symptom appears when "as a result of repression the intended course of the excitatory process in the id does not occur at all; the ego succeeds in inhibiting or deflecting it" (Freud, 1926, p. 91). This ego, which is in a somewhat privileged position in relation to perception and thus consciousness of the outside world, "wards off internal and external dangers alike along identical lines" (Freud, 1926, p. 92) by means of a flight. Whilst the external stimuli are met with bodily movements (for example, you may 'run away'), an internal unwelcomed process will be met with repression. The ego will withdraw the cathexis emerging off an instinct (as the translation goes, or the 'drive') that is going to be repressed and will 'employ' "that cathexis for the purpose of releasing unpleasure (anxiety)" (Freud, 1926, p. 93). Therefore, with this mechanism, Freud supersedes his earlier account of an automatic transformation of what is repressed into anxiety, bringing it into the realm of the ego, which allows for a more complex mapping of the subject, their being in the world, their bodily being in the world and stimuli of all orders. The libidinal excess from the drive and from reality-resting are routed by a gatekeeping ego, which manages the rhythm of excess in light of a possible dissolution of the ego's stability. Anxiety, therefore, is a by-product of the Id.

Otto Rank's then contemporary theory of the trauma of birth as one of the early universal 'mnemic symbols' for anxiety also leaves space for other traumatic experiences and the sexual act to act as such symbols—which appears in Freud's earlier writings on this topic. Freud writes: "Anxiety is not newly created in repression; it is reproduced as an affective state in accordance with an already existing mnemic image. If we go further and enquire into the origin of that anxiety—and of affects in general—we shall be leaving the realm of pure psychology and entering the borderland of physiology" (Freud, 1926, p. 93). Rank's theories, that Freud was writing in contrast with, suggested that birth was the universal traumatic experience and the nucleus of the neuroses. However, "Freud's examination shows that this cannot be the case. A child's anxiety-potential increases, not decreases after birth" (Mitchell, 1974, p. 81). What is particularly interesting at this point is the connection Freud makes with affect as a kind of blueprint that gets repeated. He writes: "Affective states have become incorporated in the mind as precipitates of primaeval traumatic experiences, and when a similar situation occurs they are revived like mnemic symbols" (Freud, 1926, p. 93). As we can see, affect thus appears in this piece as a repetition without difference; here we see anxiety as reproducing 'being' and hardly opening into new 'becomings'.

Repression being the activating mechanism of symptom-formation and anxiety, according to Freud's logic, remains slightly puzzling, especially in regard to its relation with the super-ego. This leaves Freud with an open-ended understanding that there are primal repressions and an 'after-pressure', which could be perhaps demarcated by the emergence of the super-ego; nonetheless, in small children, who are pre-Oedipal, there is, as he sees, still intense anxiety.

When repression fails, "the instinctual impulse has found a substitute in spite of repression, but a substitute which is very much reduced, displaced and inhibited and which is no longer recognizable as a satisfaction" (Freud, 1926, p. 95). In trying to satisfy a drive via such substitutive process (which is the dynamic of symptoms, in a general sense), the repressive mechanism "is forced to expend itself in making alterations in the subject's own body and is not permitted to impinge upon the external world. It must not be transformed into action" (Freud, 1926, p. 95). The 'internalisation' of the effect of repression *en route* to become anxiety is explained as follows: "As we know, in repression the ego is operating under the influence of external reality and therefore it debars the substitutive process from having any effect upon that reality" (Freud, 1926, p. 95). The ego at first struggles against this newly emerged symptom, as if trying to get rid of a 'foreign body'; however, a secondary, and, as Freud sees it, more complicated process takes place subsequently, that of a 'conciliation' to the point of enjoyment—as Lacan would phrase it—with this symptom. Freud writes:

> Being of a peaceable disposition it [the ego] would like to incorporate the symptom and make it part of itself. It is from the symptom itself that the trouble comes. For the symptom, being the true substitute for and derivative of the repressed impulse, carries on the role of the latter; it continually renews its demands for satisfaction and thus obliges the ego in its turn to give the signal of unpleasure and put itself in a posture of defence. (Freud, 1926, p. 100)

This 'signal of unpleasure' is anxiety. With the introduction of the 'signal', following what I presented in the Introduction, anxiety appears as fundamentally a psychosocial phenomenon, comprising a subject beyond itself. Freud reworks yet another of his earlier ideas, that which argued that anxiety is produced by repression. By dissecting neurosis through the cases of phobia in Little Hans and the Wolf Man, pointing at each case's symptom and inhibitions whilst working on their castration anxiety, Freud elaborates that "the majority of phobias go back to an anxiety of this kind felt by the ego in regard to the demands of the libido. It is always the ego's attitude of anxiety which is the primary thing and which sets repression going. Anxiety never arises from repressed libido" (Freud, 1926, p. 109). Anxiety, thus, "is produced from the libidinal cathexis of the instinctual impulses" (Freud, 1926, p. 110), slightly different to what he suggested in his early theories.

Conversion Hysterias and obsessional neurosis bring, on their turn, another layer to Freud's understanding of the symptom in relation to the logic of satisfaction and the 'agency' of the ego, the id and the super-ego over one another. In obsessional neurosis, the tendency in symptom-formation "is to give ever greater room to substitutive satisfaction at the expense of frustration. Symptoms which once stood for a restriction of the ego come later on to represent satisfactions as well, thanks to the ego's inclination to synthesis, and it is quite clear that this second meaning gradually becomes the more important of the two" (Freud, 1926, p. 118). The ego is then reduced to the role of satisfying the symptom, as Freud writes: "The over-acute conflict between id and superego which has dominated the illness from the very beginning may assume such extensive proportions that the ego, unable to carry out its office of mediator, can undertake nothing which is not drawn into the sphere of that conflict" (Freud, 1926, p. 118). This riddle brought to light from cases of phobia, obsessive neurosis and conversion hysterias is somewhat problematised in the following pages, when Freud brings up the remarkable hypothesis that castration anxiety lays in the backdrop of anxiety in general. Juliet Mitchell (1974) argues, in her influential *Psychoanalysis and Feminism*, that it is in this essay when Freud reformulates his theories of anxiety, that he "changed not the nature but the connotations and scope of the theory of castration. Anxiety precedes the fear of castration; it is a red-light warning of a possible danger" (Mitchell, 1974, p. 81). Castration, as a cornerstone of subjectivity within the Oedipal metaphor, as I will reach in what follows, is a problematic point of criticism from feminist scholars to the mental life assumed by psychoanalysis.[1] Whilst the Freudian subject is indeed psychosocial—rather than solely biological or individualised, as mainstream practices of psy will have it—this subject is still anchored in a type of subjective alienation in which the 'moral' of the Oedipal father is internalised in a guarantee to an affective modulation, crystallising patriarchy as a means to manage the excessiveness of the drive—a view that is not sufficiently challenged by even some feminist contemporary psychoanalysts such as Gherovici (2018).

According to Freud, in phobias, the relation to castration anxiety is rather straightforward: "As soon as the ego recognises the danger of castration it gives the signal of anxiety and inhibits through the pleasure-unpleasure agency (in a way which we cannot as yet understand) the impending cathectic process in the id" (Freud, 1926, p. 125). In this case of phobia, the ego is successful in its 'solution' to anxiety, avoiding it by avoiding the 'object' where it was displaced to or through the very inhibitory symptom. What Freud suggests, making this 'simple' economic equation more sophisticated, is that the danger in phobia towards which the ego is giving a signal is the danger of castration, in a manner that is no different to a 'realistic anxiety'—when there is something 'real' threatening the subject—the difference however being "that its content remains unconscious and only becomes conscious in the form of a distortion" (Freud, 1926, p. 126). Similarly, in obsessional neurosis, a danger is also being 'solved', but the difference here is that "the danger-situation from which the ego must get away is the hostility of the superego" (Freud, 1926, p. 128), an internalised danger, not external. This 'threat' on the

[1] As early as 1975, the anthropologist Gayle Rubin writes of psychoanalysis' use for feminism, in the essay 'Traffic in Women', famously calling psychoanalysis a 'failed' type of feminism. For Rubin, "Psychoanalysis contains a unique set of concepts for understanding men, women, and sexuality. It is a theory of sexuality in human society. Most importantly, psychoanalysis provides a description of the mechanisms by which the sexes are divided and deformed, of how bisexual, androgynous infants are transformed into boys and girls. Psychoanalysis is a feminist theory *manqué*" (Rubin, 1975, p. 185). Heleieth Saffioti, a pioneer Brazilian Marxist Feminist, had already published in 1969 a similar critique of Freudian psychoanalysis, stressing that Freud's theory of femininity validated anatomic difference as anchor of a patriarchal domination between two sexes (Saffioti, 1975).

ego parting from a scrutinising superego is also 'felt' as real and also derives from castration, but in this case it becomes what Freud calls 'moral anxiety'.

So far, what Freud offers on the topic of anxiety is that anxiety is, be it in cases of phobia, hysteria or obsessional neurosis, a 'reaction' to some 'situation of danger', and it becomes apparent "by the ego's doing something to avoid that situation or to withdraw from it" (Freud, 1926, p. 128). Whilst anxiety itself is not a symptom, but an unwanted affect that serves as a signal to this imminent danger, "symptoms are created so as to avoid a danger-situation whose presence has been signalled by the generation of anxiety" (Freud, 1926, p. 129). The danger situation, the threat, to which anxiety is a signal of, is lined by castration, which, for Freud at this point, can be identified in various instances, from separation to death, all of which present a danger to the integrity of the ego. He writes: "I am therefore inclined to adhere to the view that the fear of death should be regarded as analogous to the fear of castration and that the situation to which the ego is reacting is one of being abandoned by the protecting super-ego—the powers of destiny—so that it has no longer any safeguard against all the dangers that surround it" (Freud, 1926, p. 130). What we see here is this danger of fragmentation, of an annihilation of the unifying or 'stable'—even if by an illusion of stability—sense of self as the basis of anxiety. This characteristic underlies the of anxiety as a vibration, as it will become clearer as we move along. This is also precisely the grounds for anxiety Lacan will be working with, situating the subject as bound to the Other, in a position lacking of any autonomy, which is at the foundations for his theories on anxiety. Evidently, the choice of the word 'castration' and its reverberations with 'lack' within a phallic matrix of subjectivity are far from unproblematic from feminist lenses.

For Freud, the 'manifestation' of anxiety is particular to the body, to specific 'physical sensations' that are here pointed as mostly respiratory, connected to the heart and motor in their discharge. In short, anxiety is linked to "(1) a specific character of unpleasure, (2) acts of discharge and (3) perceptions of those acts" (Freud, 1926, pp. 132–133). And it is precisely in the way anxiety is characterised through the acts of discharge connected to it and how such acts are perceived that anxiety differs from other kinds of 'un-pleasures'. Freud even offers the specific examples of pain and mourning, that can be similar, yet diverge in their 'discharge', for "anxiety is based upon an increase of excitation which on the one hand produces the character of unpleasure and on the other finds relief through the acts of discharge" (Freud, 1926, p. 133). Despite its remarking physiological characteristics, which Freud mentions as an increase in excitation that produces unpleasure and at the same time finds a path of discharge; there is more to anxiety than this very physiology. The unconscious is also highly associated in this 'specificity' of anxiety, once there is a specific 'temporality' of anxiety brought together by the very 'marks' it leaves on the subject and their experience. This 'line' or 'trail' of anxiety is, Freud supposes, connected to a 'model' experience that is reproduced through the anxious feeling, this initial experience "contained the necessary conditions for such an increase of excitation and a discharge along particular paths, and that from this circumstance the unpleasure of anxiety receives its specific character" (Freud, 1926, p. 133). One of such early experiences is the trauma of birth. Whilst Freud acknowledges that some biological observations with non-mammals can possibly refute the trauma of birth theory, it nonetheless cannot be so easily discarded in relation to the human experience, and what follows from this assumption would be the questioning of 'why' anxiety. What would be its function, presuming there is any? "The answer seems to be obvious and convincing: anxiety arose originally as a reaction to a state of *danger* and it is reproduced whenever a state of that kind recurs" (Freud, 1926, p. 134).

Instead of the trauma of birth in the way Rank has proposed, Freud sees birth and the subsequent developments in small children as allowing for a 'primal anxiety' which is linked to the fear of object loss. This fear of object loss and anxiety are, however, enveloped in the same danger-signal logic. Freud suggests earlier that this involves this initial danger, a possibility raised in the infant's awareness that without the 'mother' it can vanish without care, nourishment, etc., all of which is 'processed' by the infant as a satisfaction-unsatisfied-unpleasure state. This growing tension that emerges with need and the state of non-satisfaction that sees stimuli accumulating to the point of unpleasure sees infants unable to master this tension physically or discharge it, "analogous to the experience of being born" (Freud, 1926, p. 137), giving rise to anxiety in relation to this very 'danger'. Only when the baby is able to process this danger as linked to the presence of the mother that her absence becomes a danger itself.

Yet, an early infant anxiety, this primary anxiety and the fear of loss are also analogous to what happens later on, when castration becomes the danger, when the phallic phase is reached, as "in this case the danger is of being separated from one's genitals" (Freud, 1926, p. 139). The genital, particularly the penis, of high narcissistic value, as Freud paraphrases from Ferenczi, is linked with the fantasy of it being what could once again unite the child with the mother. In castration, "being deprived of it [the phallus] amounts to a renewed separation from her, and this in its turn means being helplessly exposed to an unpleasurable tension due to instinctual need, as was the case at birth" (Freud, 1926, p. 139). At this point Freud introduces the problematic riddle of sexual difference to his theory of anxiety, which, as I will discuss in what follows, is important in the formulation of a psychosocial approach to this affect that does not rely on Oedipal sexual difference as the anchor of subjectivity.

For Freud, with the subsequent refinement of perception and psychic activities, the fear of loss of the mother and castration are followed by the super-ego, when the latter is 'installed' as a 'depersonalisation' of the parental figure/agency that once allowed for castration. When the super-ego is installed as part of the psychic structure, a type of anxiety emerges which is social and Freud calls 'moral anxiety'. Subsequently, the ego will signal with anxiety when the 'disapproval' from the super-ego becomes prominent. And here, in this complex state of anxiety in relation to the super-ego, a foundation for the Lacanian anxiety and the desire of the Other is laid down: "The final transformation which the fear of the super-ego undergoes is, it seems [to me], the fear of death (or fear for life) which is a fear of the super-ego projected on to the powers of destiny" (Freud, 1926, p. 140). Or, as Lacan asks, in Italian: *Che vuoi?*

Avoiding danger, removing oneself from the possibility of it, the reactions to this danger are closely linked to anxiety and of course the question of what are these dangers and the place they occupy in one's psychic structure is the next question, that is addressed on a tangent. Freud moves to the end of this essay by summarising the different 'stages' in life as per how one is situated to face one's anxiety, a process that culminates with negotiations over the process of 'being in the world' in the most direct sense. There is a justification of a moral internalisation and the affect of anxiety as correlate, not to mention the, yet again, focus on the 'boy's' psychosexual development.

> In early infancy the individual is really not equipped to master psychically the large sums of excitation that reach him whether from without or from within. Again, at a certain period of life his most important interest really is that the people he is dependent on should not withdraw their loving care of him. Later on in his boyhood, when he feels that his father is a powerful rival in regard to his mother and becomes aware of his own aggressive inclinations towards him and of his sexual intentions towards his mother, he really is justified in being afraid of his father; and his fear of being punished by him can find expression through phylogenetic reinforcement in the fear of being castrated. Finally, as he enters into social relationships, it really is necessary for him to be afraid of his super-ego, to have a conscience; and the absence of that factor would give rise to severe conflicts, dangers and so on. (Freud, 1926, pp. 146–147)

This 'line' is not particularly 'linear' in everyone's experiences, as a person can get caught in an earlier manner of dealing with the excess stimuli and "remain infantile in their behaviour in regard to danger and do not overcome determinants of anxiety which have grown out of date" (Freud, 1926, p. 146). That would characterise neurosis and also offer light on the quantitative aspects of this economy of stimuli in the dynamics of repression. Repression, repetition and anxiety form a cycle of excesses and remainders operating in a somewhat non-organised circuit, propelled by the interplay of control and excess of libido so vividly evidenced in the production of anxiety.

Sexual difference as well as moral anxiety and castration are for Juliet Mitchell (1974) central themes for a feminist engagement with psychoanalysis, once they are intrinsically linked with the debate of the Oedipus Complex. Anxiety, thus, has a feminine imprint in Freudian thought, as she explains:

> The anxiety caused by the mother going can be resolved by understanding that she will come back [...]. The point is that this anxiety does not (any more than does the anxiety of birth), involve socially unacceptable ideas.

> On the other hand, the incestuous desire for the mother that then arises does involve the forbidden. Now, anxiety comes into play to suggest fear of castration if these incestuous ideas are not abandoned. [...] If the castration complex is not adequately resolved—and that means the possibility of castration in not symbolically accepted, then the Oedipus complex is not shattered and aspects of its irresolution will recur in later neurosis. (Mitchell, 1974, p. 82)

Freud, through the function of the phallus (in the evident description of patriarchy present in his theory of psychosexual development), connects narcissism and the Oedipus complex—or a modulation of desire within a politically situated family drama, as Deleuze and Guattari (1983) will denounce in *Anti-Oedipus*—with the concept of castration. This model of positing sexual difference thus relied on the artifice of anxiety, once a fear of castration would, for a little boy, be expressed through an outburst of anxiety, such as seen in the case of Little Hans. Mitchell writes:

> Freud gave a number of reasons for the value attached to the phallus [...]. Having incorporated it into the concept of narcissism—its ownership is crucial to the nature of the ego being formed, or rather its loss would be an immense blow for the narcissistic ego—Freud had to recognise the distinction between the sexes in this respect. This recognition, and the diverse role of the castration complex, led him, in the second half of the twenties and thirties to a reassessment of the Oedipus complex and from there to the development of his theories of femininity and the pre-Oedipal narcissistic stage. (Mitchell, 1974, p. 88)

Lacan will make castration anxiety even more central to his theory of this affect. Castration and the phallic law, as well as a positioning of the subject on the side of 'having it' or 'lacking it' in a Symbolic and Imaginary form, are the grounds for his theory of sexual difference. What Juliet Mitchell observed, so early in the encounter between psychoanalysis and feminism, and what she argues in *Psychoanalysis and Feminism*, is that Freud's theory of anxiety, which unfolds through lack, loss and separation, is utilised to account for a type of castration (the 'castration complex'), for when castration is already there ('femininity'). Anxiety, thus, is a feminist issue.

As we have seen so far, in this paper, Freud makes several changes to his previous views on the topic of anxiety, taking into account his works in other texts as mentioned before such as 'Beyond the Pleasure Principle', 1920, and 'The Ego and the Id', 1923. Anxiety, by 1926, then, is more complex than an overwhelming excess of libido finding its 'way out'; it now passes through the mental apparatus, mobilising the body accordingly, in much less 'pre-arranged' zig zags, once the Id and also repression come to negotiate stimuli, protections, symptoms and remainders. The ego is the 'seat' but also the 'source' of anxiety—an assertion that Lacan would challenge in his take on the subject, taking it away from the ego. Rank's work on the trauma of birth as a 'prototype' to anxiety was also worked over, raising the central discussion around what is perceived as a situation of danger, a threat to the ego, and not only neurotic or realistic anxieties but also moral anxiety. The existence of an 'original' situation of danger was circumvented until Freud was able to reach the heart of the question in the identification of the factor of a 'threat to the ego'.

Anxiety as 'signal', as it has been conceptualised in this paper, also comes close to 'fear', nonetheless Freud offers a very precise clarification of the difference between the two. Again, this is a point that Lacan will pick up later in relation to anxiety and the 'lack of the lack', subverting Freudian logic. To Freud, "anxiety [Angst] has an unmistakable relation to expectation: it is anxiety about something. It has a quality of indefiniteness and lack of object. In precise speech we use the word 'fear' [Furcht] rather than 'anxiety' [Angst] if it has found an object" (Freud, 1926, p. 165). Having 'something' to be anxious 'about' brings up the question of the nature of this 'something', of it being 'real' or 'not real', and in this paper Freud insists that something is 'real' as long as it feels as such to the subject. In this sense, a bearing on 'material reality' is not what defines what is a 'realistic' of neurotic anxiety, rather, the external (as in an external object) or internal (instinctual/drive-related) 'nature of this sources' of anxiety, both share the same 'realistic basis'.

## New Introductory Lectures on Psycho-Analysis: Lecture XXXII Anxiety and Instinctual Life, 1933

Written in 1932 and published the following year, Freud's *New Introductory Lectures* series was never delivered, rather, printed straight away in 1933, covering a number of topics that crossed psychoanalysis. The lecture on 'Anxiety and Instinctual Life', the last of his pieces dedicated specifically to the theme of anxiety, sets off by promising updates but nevertheless no real 'final' answers in regard to the riddle of anxiety. The text, in the first half, in particular, when recapping the previous lecture on the same topic, Lecture XXV from 1917, and updating its findings, is very much in line with the contributions found in 'Inhibitions, Symptoms and Anxiety', pointing at an anxiety as signal to a situation of danger; a danger deriving from a traumatic experience and an anxiety formed around the fear of castration and its repercussions.

Freud departs from what is known about anxiety by that point, that it is "an affective estate—that is to say, a combination of certain feelings in the pleasure-unpleasure series with the corresponding innervations of discharge and a perception of them, but probably also the precipitate of a particular important event, incorporated by inheritance" (Freud, 1933, p. 81). Anxiety had a sort of 'footprint' on the psyche-body that would see itself resonating in future experiences of anxiety. Another point raised still in 1917 was in relation to the different 'types' of anxiety: neurotic and realistic, and their origin and process. Whilst the latter seems to be clearer to understanding, as a response to an external threat and the preparedness towards it, the former, by his account, was still left slightly up in the air in 1917. However, the 1926 essay deals with this difference in more detail.

One key aspect that is now clearer in relation to anxiety in cases of hysteria and neurosis is the mechanism of repression, that by now, towards the later years of Freud's life, is more refined than what was offered in early texts. By 1932 he was already working over his second topographical model of the psychic apparatus, and the id, ego and super-ego come to function as dynamic agencies of the psyche with more clarity. In regard to anxiety and repression, our understanding can benefit

> if we separate what happens to the idea that has to be repressed from what happens to the quota of libido attaching to it. It is the idea which is subjected to repression and which may be distorted to the point of being unrecognizable; but its quota of affect is regularly transformed into anxiety—and this is so whatever the nature of the affect may be, whether it is aggressiveness or love. (Freud, 1933, p. 83)

In light of this transformation, Freud reminds us of previous works in linking symptom and anxiety—a correlation that becomes confused at times in the 1926 work, precisely because they "represent and replace each other" (Freud, 1933, p. 83) in different case scenarios. Therefore, "it seems, indeed, that the generation of anxiety is the earlier and the formation of symptoms the later of the two, as though the symptoms are created in order to avoid the outbreak of the anxiety state" (Freud, 1933, p. 84). Another point clarified on this occasion is that what one is really afraid of in cases of neurotic anxiety and realistic anxiety is their own libido, and the difference here would be that in neurotic anxiety "danger is internal instead of an external one and that it is not consciously recognised" (Freud, 1933, p. 84). This 're-employment' of libido in anxiety and the fact that it may be replaced by a symptom that is 'physically bound' is what gains more consistency in this current presentation, once, as Freud points out, it is in the interplay between id, ego and super-ego that we can grasp further what is the Freudian contribution to the riddle of anxiety.

The ego being, as he previously established, the 'seat of anxiety', does not mean that despite anxiety not being 'in' the id, for instance, that these other psychic agencies do not exercise any impact on the formation of anxiety. Quite the contrary, as Freud elaborated in the 1926 piece, there is a centrality of castration anxiety that can be read over different cases and at different moments in life of any individual. He related the 'fear of castration' to a sense of helplessness, lack of autonomy and a threat to the subject. Yet, so far the Freudian subject of anxiety has been—despite the account of hysteria—much focused on a presupposed 'male/masculine' individual. Here Freud for once differentiates castration in the possible implications it has over sexual difference, whilst still keeping to the 'findings' of the work on the previous decades:

> Fear of castration is not, of course, the only motive for repression: indeed, it finds no place in women, for though they have a castration complex they cannot have a fear of being castrated. Its place is taken in their sex by a fear of loss of love, which is evidently a later prolongation of the infant's anxiety if it finds its mother absent. You will realise how real a situation of danger is indicated by this anxiety. If a mother is absent or has withdrawn her love from her child, it is no longer sure of the satisfaction of its needs and is perhaps exposed to the most distressing feelings of tension. (Freud, 1933, p. 87)

What is interesting here is that Rank's trauma of birth and the centrality over this separation from the mother, instead of a centrality in castration, could somehow hint at a less Oedipal sexual difference in the foundations of anxiety. Yet, as Freud dismisses this claim of the centrality of the trauma of birth, we are left with anxiety as a riddle that seats in the ego but is mobilised by the id and the super-ego as well and mobilising the body in its turn through a path that, in this account, relies on the Oedipal structure. What we can also read into this centrality of castration is a problematic infantilisation of women/femininity, once he posits that:

> The danger of psychical helplessness fits the stage of the ego's early immaturity; the danger of loss of an object (or loss of love) fits the lack of self-sufficiency in the first years of childhood; the danger of being castrated fits the phallic phase; and finally fear of the super-ego, which assumes a special position, fits the period of latency. In the course of development the old determinants of anxiety should be dropped, since the situations of danger corresponding to them have lost their importance owing to the strengthening of the ego. But this only occurs most incompletely. Many people are unable to surmount the fear of loss of love; they never become sufficiently independent of other people's love and in this respect carry on their behaviour as infants. (Freud, 1933, p. 88)

Through this logic Freud explains how neurotics are held onto this early, infantile relation to danger, not being able to ingress in the phallic phase that entails a 'getting over' the fear of being 'left', just as for women. Women, for not being able to enter the Oedipal phase as such, and neurotics are stuck in this infantilised state. An obvious testament to Freud's patriarchal views—which I add to what has been elaborated by Juliet Mitchell (1974) on the topic, as mentioned above.

Another key aspect of Freud's late theory of anxiety is its relation to repression. Whilst at first it was thought that repression generated anxiety, we now understand that it is the other way around, as previously mentioned. Anxiety, therefore, is located in the interplay between ego and id. Such ego and id relation in anxiety only becomes clear after the 1923 text, substituting the visual model of vessels of quantities Freud proposed in the 'Project for a Scientific Psychology', outlined in 1895. The ego "makes use of an experimental cathexis and starts up the pleasure-unpleasure automatism by means of a signal of anxiety" (Freud, 1933, p. 90), which is activated on the face of the dangers of the repetition of a certain traumatic experience that would emerge if a 'call' of the id were to be attended to. Given this, anxiety and repression can go different ways. There may be an anxiety attack (which is when the ego withdraws completely from what Freud calls this 'objectionable excitation' it is alerting against) or the ego may offer a counter-balance, an anticathexis that will be joined by the reserved energy of the repressed impulse resulting in a symptom.

Signal anxiety 'sets in action' the pleasure-unpleasure principle impact of repression, transforming what goes on in the id, or '*instinctual/drive* impulses' that belong there. Freud offers different scenarios to what happens in the id through repression. "In some cases the repressed *instinctual* impulse may retain its libidinal cathexis, and may persist in the id unchanged, although subject to constant pressure from the ego" (Freud, 1933, p. 92). At other times this 'instinctual impulse' vanishes leaving only a trace of libido, of energy, that is 'diverted' thereafter—which he posits as being the case when the Oedipus complex is well resolved. Another option would be for "a regression of the libidinal organisation to an earlier stage. This can, of course, only occur in the id, and if it occurs it will be under the influence of the same conflict which was introduced by the signal of anxiety" (Freud, 1933, p. 92).

Quantities of tension that cannot be dealt with, which are overwhelming to the consistency of the subject, are still the backbone of anxiety. This includes signal anxiety, where "what is feared, what is the object of the anxiety, is invariably the emergence of a traumatic moment, which cannot be dealt with by the normal rules of the pleasure principle" (Freud, 1933, p. 94). Therefore, anxiety is almost a secondary process that has to have an initial point at a previous experience, a rule maintained even when it is a case of anxiety neurosis "owing to somatic damage to the sexual function" (Freud, 1933, p. 94). A fresh contribution in this text then is this short observation that supersedes the 1926 text, stating that "we shall no longer maintain that it is the libido itself that is turned into anxiety in such cases [of anxiety neurosis linked to the bodily sexual function]" (Freud, 1933, p. 94). In summary, Freud offers "a twofold origin of anxiety—one as a direct consequence of the traumatic moment and the other as a signal threatening a repetition of such a moment" (Freud, 1933, p. 94). And in so doing, he moves psychoanalysis away from its cruder focus on the sexual drive and towards the matter of an overwhelming threat to the consistency of the ego.

Yet again, Freud's view of anxiety is that it is a central affect to 'normal' experience and that it has a function. By functioning as a signal to a threat to the stability of the ego, anxiety is able to establish itself as a 'compass' in the map of the treatment (Miller, 2007). It is by going through the clues of anxiety that we can get in touch to what is anchoring one's ego. Whilst some clinical approaches (from mainstream biologist psychiatry to certain orientations in psychoanalysis) might find value in strengthening the ego's mechanisms of defence (from some psychoanalytic schools to forms of counselling and psychotherapy that are humanistic, or 'person-centred'), or one's 'ideal of oneself' (think here of CBT, Positive Psychology and wellness, in general), a Freudo-Lacanian practice will lead towards disputing the very illusion that the ego consists on. Anxiety is then the guiding principle of this practice; and if one has to be less anxious, the solution is to make the ego less stiff and a little more malleable. Instead of a stranger, anxiety is deeply entangled into the Freudian subject.

## The Trail of Anxiety in Freud

The very final systematic account of anxiety in Freudian writing appears in one of his last written pieces, before passing away in London. In 'An Outline of Psychoanalysis', from 1938, his later ideas about the id, the ego and the functions and dynamics of anxiety are expressed. We quite clearly see anxiety as a negotiation between these psychic agencies, operating as a threshold of overwhelming tension and the movement of preservation of integrity. The ego appears as a gatekeeper, guaranteeing an adaptation to the 'world', against both internal and external dangers of annihilation of the subject. The id, in this final account, appears as a still mysterious and charged psychic sphere that is directly connected with the body, the drive and perception. Freud writes:

> The id, cut off from the external world, has a world of perception of its own. It detects with extraordinary acuteness certain changes in its interior, especially oscillations in the tension of its instinctual needs, and these changes become conscious as feelings in the pleasure-unpleasure series. It is hard to say, to be sure, by what means and with the help of what sensory terminal organs these perceptions come about. But it is an established fact that self-perceptions—coenaesthetic feelings and feelings of pleasure-unpleasure—govern the passage of events in the id with despotic force. (Freud, 1938, p. 198)

This overwhelming flow of pleasure-unpleasure is then channelled through the activity of the ego, guided by 'the sensations of anxiety'. In Freud's words: "The ego has set itself the task of self-preservation, which the id appears to neglect. It [the ego] makes use of the sensations of anxiety as a signal to give a warning of dangers that threaten its integrity" (Freud, 1938, p. 199). It is interesting that Freud's development of his theory of anxiety as a signal of an imminent threat first starts with a focus on realistic dangers, which are dangers to the body and to life. He then moves on to dangers that are more subjective, related to the ego, to the preservation of some integrity and a sense of 'self' that is guaranteed and stabilised through the ego's activities. Post-Freudian psychoanalysis—especially in the context of the several Jewish analysts that escaped Nazi persecution in Europe during and around the period of WWII—grows in the United States into a further preoccupation with these promises of stability conferred to a well-functioning ego. Adaptation and strengthening the ego's defences become central to the work developed by Anna Freud in the 1940s in Britain and by Ego-Psychology in the United States (Frosh, 1987). In France, Lacan puts this into question, twisting the roles of the id and ego. Freud's '*Wo Es War, Soll Ich Werden*' becomes "Where it was, I must come into being" (Lacan, 1957 [2006], p. 435). Anxiety, as an affect of sensations that at once overwhelm and inform the ego, assumes a central and intriguing role in subjectivity. It can at the same time paralyse and cause suffering, whilst it may point at new horizons, opening up the gates of the id beyond the limits of the 'illusion' of the ego.

This view of the function of anxiety is, therefore, contrary to the hegemonic psychiatric nosology, where, instead, the goal is to eliminate anxiety altogether, keeping any 'sense of self' unexamined. From this perspective, the Freudian view of anxiety already hints at a possible 'becoming' away from a frozen 'being'. In doing so, the Freudian theories of anxiety open the way to an understanding of anxiety as a 'vibration', or as an affect of the order of excess, beyond the delineation of the individual.

In the 1920s and early 1930s, there is a strong reliance on the Oedipal myth and a subsequent formulation of castration anxiety that anchors the psychoanalytic understanding of sexual difference. However, what this detailed close reading of this archive has revealed is the potential of the 'unbound' character of anxiety found in the pre-psychoanalytic texts, the 1917 paper and the 1938 text. In these occasions, Freud does not rely on the Oedipal model so strongly, rather connecting anxiety to (1) excessive libido and (2) the id. The early energetic model of psyche-soma will map anxiety into a dynamic of excessive libidinal pressure that will result in anxiety. The locus of libido is the Id. When Freud, in 1938, say that the id "has a world of perception of its own" (Freud, 1938, p. 198) he leaves a door open for an understanding of affect that extends beyond the 'I' (ego, Ich), beyond morality/internalised culture or modulations of desire (superego). The id, thus, is crossed by perceptions of what extends beyond oneself, which produce pressure onto the ego, an activity such that Freud sees as anxiety. If anxiety is then seen as a production in the 'I' that echoes an accumulation, or a flow of libido imprinted upon the Id but accumulated not just through the drive, but also through this 'perception' capacity of the Id, then anxiety is an affect that vibrates between a 'being' (the ego/superego consistencies of the subject) and 'becomings'—or the effects of the flows perceived in the Id of what extends beyond the 'I' and might put the very consistency of the 'I' at risk.

In this chapter, a close reading of Freud's systematic delineations of the grounds of anxiety allows us to rescue two main pillars of his theory. These are first, the rescuing of Freud's very early account of anxiety that is not reliant on an Oedipal understanding of the subject. Secondly, the function of anxiety as a signal for the insistence of ego-activity in preserving a sense of reality. Lacan will formulate a theory of anxiety as an affect that marks an encounter with the Real that takes these two pillars of Freudian theory further. He will, specifically, problematise the promise of a strong ego in a theory of anxiety as 'excess'.

Freud's very early work, in the nineteenth century, addresses the question of anxiety as an excess that is not bound to symbolisation or to Oedipal function. What we have seen is a dynamic relation between the 'libidinal flow' and 'representatives', or ideas, in Freud's model of psyche-soma. A 'conversion' takes place when the surplus tension of the drive cannot find sufficient or adequate grounds in the frameworks enveloping it. In the case of hysteria, for example, there is an established tradition of feminist thinking of this mode of conversion under the lenses of hysteria and hysteric symptoms as a form of social protest against a patriarchal arrangement (from Cixous, 1976 and Mitchell, 2000 to Webster, 2018 among several others). In Lacanian parlance it would be a case of the explicit limits of the Symbolic and relation to the Real in hysteria as well as in anxiety. In anxiety a 'conversion' takes place moving the Real of the body that finds no place in experience. In other words, the phenomenological body of the subject in culture as experiencing the resonances of a chaotic and excessive energetic flow is evident in Freud's very early account of anxiety. This is foundational to delineating anxiety as a 'vibration'.

## References


Berrios, G. E. (1996). *The History of Mental Symptoms: Descriptive Psychopathology Since the Nineteenth Century*. Cambridge University Press.

Cixous, H. (1976). The Laugh of the Medusa. *Signs, 1*(4, Summer), 875–893.

Deleuze, G., & Guattari, F. (1983). *Anti-Oedipus – Capitalism and Schizophrenia*. University of Minnesota Press.

Freud, S. (1892). Draft B from Extracts from the Fliess Papers. In *The Standard Edition of the Complete Psychological Works of Sigmund Freud, Volume I (1886-1899): Pre-Psycho-Analytic Publications and Unpublished Drafts* (pp. 179–184).

Freud, S. (1894a, June 6). Draft E. How Anxiety Originates. In *The Complete Letters of Sigmund Freud to Wilhelm Fliess, 1887-1904* (pp. 78–83).

Freud, S. (1894b). On The Grounds for Detaching a Particular Syndrome from Neurasthenia Under The Description 'Anxiety Neurosis'. In *The Standard Edition of the Complete Psychological Works of Sigmund Freud, Volume III (1893-1899): Early Psycho-Analytic Publications* (pp. 85–115).

Freud, S. (1895). A Reply to Criticisms of My Paper on Anxiety Neurosis. In *The Standard Edition of the Complete Psychological Works of Sigmund Freud, Volume III (1893-1899): Early Psycho-Analytic Publications* (pp. 119–139).

Freud, S. (1917). Introductory Lectures on Psycho-Analysis. In *The Standard Edition of the Complete Psychological Works of Sigmund Freud, Volume XVI (1916-1917): Introductory Lectures on Psycho-Analysis (Part III)* (pp. 241–463).

Freud, S. (1920). Beyond the Pleasure Principle. In *The Standard Edition of the Complete Psychological Works of Sigmund Freud, Volume XVIII (1920-1922): Beyond the Pleasure Principle, Group Psychology and Other Works* (pp. 1–64).

Freud, S. (1923). The Ego and the Id. In *The Standard Edition of the Complete Psychological Works of Sigmund Freud, Volume XIX (1923-1925): The Ego and the Id and Other Works* (pp. 1–66).

Freud, S. (1925). An Autobiographical Study. In *The Standard Edition of the Complete Psychological Works of Sigmund Freud, Volume XX (1925-1926): An Autobiographical Study, Inhibitions, Symptoms and Anxiety, The Question of Lay Analysis and Other Works* (pp. 1–74).

Freud, S. (1926). Inhibitions, Symptoms and Anxiety. In *The Standard Edition of the Complete Psychological Works of Sigmund Freud, Volume XX (1925-1926): An Autobiographical Study, Inhibitions, Symptoms and Anxiety, The Question of Lay Analysis and Other Works* (pp. 75–176).

Freud, S. (1933). Lecture XXXII Anxiety and Instinctual Life. New Introductory Lectures on Psycho-Analysis. In *The Standard Edition of the Complete Psychological Works of Sigmund Freud, Volume XXII (1932-1936): New Introductory Lectures on Psycho-Analysis and Other Works* (pp. 1–182).

Freud, S. (1938). An Outline of Psycho-Analysis. In *The Standard Edition of the Complete Psychological Works of Sigmund Freud, Volume XXIII (1937-1939): Moses and Monotheism, An Outline of Psycho-Analysis and Other Works* (pp. 139–208).

Frosh, S. (1987). *The Politics of Psychoanalysis*. Macmillan.

Gherovici, P. (2018). Anxious? Castration Is the Solution! *Psychoanalytic Inquiry, 38*(1), 83–90.

Lacan, J. (1957). The Instance of the Letter in the Unconscious, or Reason Since Freud. In *Écrits:* The First Complete Edition in English (2006) [Trans. B. Fink]. W.W. Norton and Company.

Miller, J. A. (2007). *La angustia – Introducción al Seminario X de Jacques Lacan*. Gredos.

Mitchell, J. (1974). *Psychoanalysis and Feminism*. Patheon.

Mitchell, J. (2000). *Mad Men and Medusas: Reclaiming Hysteria*. Basic Books.

Rubin, G. (1975). The Traffic in Women: Notes on the 'political economy' of Sex. In R. Reiter (Ed.), *Toward and Anthropology of Women*. Monthly Review Press.

Saffioti, H. (1975). *A Mulher na Sociedade de Classes*. Vozes.

Webster, J. (2018). *Conversion Disorder: Listening to the Body in Psychoanalysis*. Columbia University Press.

# 6

# Edging the Real

After a close reading of Freud's trajectory on his theory of anxiety, we will travel into another territory and investigate Lacan's interventions on this topic. Most noticeably in his Seminar X, which focused on anxiety and departed from Freud's 1926 piece, 'Inhibitions, Symptoms and Anxiety', Lacan's understanding of this affect mobilises the register of the Real, *jouissance* and the *objet a,* central concepts in the delineation of an excessive affective vibration that I elaborate here. Lacan's anxiety brings to light an 'excess', but differently to Freud, since the latter was accounting for an economic dynamic of accumulation of tension under a logic of discharge which he understood as the central mechanism of the psychic apparatus. Lacan's 'excess' is marked in a reminder—or remainder—of singularity evidenced in anxiety, as I will be arguing in the following pages, and this has been eternalised in the often-cited passage from Seminar X that "the true substance of anxiety, is that which deceives not" (Lacan, 1962–1963 [2014], p. 76). This affirmation comes along the intellectual trajectory that marks Lacan's move beyond what he calls the register of the Imaginary, stressing its limits and bringing anxiety, thus, as


A. C. Minozzo, *Anxiety as Vibration*, Studies in the Psychosocial,
https://doi.org/10.1007/978-3-031-62856-6_6

a kind of 'proof' of the 'unreliability' of the Imaginary.[1] The year in which this seminar was delivered, 1962–1963, is also particular as Lacan's relation to the IPA was getting heated and the year came to a close with his expulsion from the international organisation in 1963 (Roudinesco, 1997). [2]With this in mind, we could argue that this split allowed Lacan more space—or increased his stubbornness—to move into his own theories, beyond his initial endeavour of a 'return to Freud'. To put it boldly, this moment of delivering Seminar X represents a turning point in Lacanian psychoanalytic theory.[3] In the seminar on anxiety, Lacan's innovation is marked by the articulations on the *objet a*, which continues in Seminar XI. This chapter will contemplate various pillars of Lacanian psychoanalytic theory, focusing on his writing up until Seminar X and the emergence of the *objet a* in relation to a structural lack, or gap, in the Lacanian subject. Mapping the development of the consistency of the subject through the theory of the mirror stage and the discussion of self-consciousness during the 1950s and 1960s, I will construct an argument with an emphasis on anxiety in relation to the Real, the body and possible readings of this 'lack' as a positive gap—or, as I am conceptualising in this cartography, a vibration—as developed in Seminar X and later seminars. It is in relation to questions of ontology, the Real and negativity that I will be distancing myself from the theories of Freud and Lacan through an engagement with Deleuze and Guattari (expanding the Real seen in Lacan's very late writings beyond the Symbolic and beyond the Oedipal metaphor), all the while trying to bring these traditions together in a 'clinically viable' concept of anxiety as vibration.

[1] The Imaginary in Lacan can be summarised as the function that offers coherence to the world 'outside' through the 'image' of the subject. Its limits, so the limits of this anchoring 'image' and 'coherence', are particularly relevant to the understanding of anxiety.

[2] Details of his break with the IPA were famously registered in the introductory section of the following seminar, Seminar XI 'The Four Fundamental Concepts of Psychoanalysis', titled '*excommunication*'.

[3] Lacan's conceptualisation of the registers of the Imaginary, the Symbolic and the Real dates from the 1940s. From the 1950s onwards, he will develop the more complex idea of the Real and in the 1970s, his later texts bring the ideas of knots, or the links between the registers. Anxiety, as Seminar X presents, marks an encounter with the register of the Real, therefore the latter has a particular importance for this research.

## Exceeding Freud

Lacan's work can be roughly divided in three phases, each lasting more or less a decade and corresponding to one of the registers of psychic life identified by him: First, the Imaginary, then the Symbolic and last, the Real. Over the course of his seminar teachings, conference presentations and writings, from the 1940s to the early 1980s, each of these registers is worked through, never in isolation or with 'privilege' over the other registers, rather, simply through a theoretical working emphasis. Why does this matter in understanding the place of 'anxiety' in Lacanian psychoanalytic work? For two reasons, both guiding this study. The most noticeable one is the place of the seminar on anxiety in this chronological line, closing the moment of the Imaginary and entering the years Lacan was mostly concerned with the Symbolic. The second reason is the 'quality of anxiety' throughout these different moments of his teachings. Early mentions of '*angoisse*' in his seminars in the 1950s are mostly concerned with Freudian case studies, from the Wolf Man in 1952–1953 or Irma's dream in 1955, to a considerable amount of attention paid to Little Hans and the writing on phobia and anxiety until the closing of the 1950s. Something will change in the seminar on anxiety and that is the beginning of Lacan's thinking of anxiety in relation to desire, a theoretical venture that carried on, despite less evident in respect to anxiety, through his very last seminars in the late 1960s and early 1970s.

Based on this sort of 'timeline', is it possible to divide Lacan's work on the topic of anxiety in about three different instances. At first, in the work that is the very early Lacan, so prior to the Seminars, there is a mention of anxiety in the 1945 paper '*Le Temps Logique*'. Here anxiety is the ontological form of a 'motivation to the conclusion', following the instant of the glance and the time for comprehending as the three evidential moments of the assertion of oneself—here already anxiety appears as a 'common' experience, rather than necessarily pathologised, in contrast with the diagnostic trend of the period. The topic is left to the side for many years, until what we could call a 'second moment' of Lacan's work on anxiety, which really focused on Freudian works, at the time of delivering Seminar II, when Lacan addresses Freud's own anxiety in the face of women when commenting on his analysis of the dream of Irma's injection. Here there is an early delineation of Lacan's work on the anxiety of the analyst, a point he will explore further in Seminar X, which is Lacan's third theory of anxiety, his most comprehensive and focused elaboration on the topic. What is missing, systematically, is a later theory of anxiety in light of his post-1963 thinking.

The Freudian base of Lacan's anxiety seminar is the 1926 text 'Inhibitions, Symptoms and Anxiety'. Lacan picks up on key Freudian concepts from 1926, signal and castration anxiety, not offering equal attention to Freud's last texts on the topic, however. What Lacan brings into Seminar X, in particular, is the fundamental tension between the subject and the Other, a relation that will reverberate with his earlier writing on the Mirror Stage and a completion of the Graph of Desire.[4] This same tension between subject and Other serves as the ground for his subsequent development of the notion of the *objet a*. It is the *objet a* that will mark the structural 'lack' of the subject and the Other, simultaneously. As we will see in the coming pages, it will be, subsequently, such 'lack' that will be reformulated in his later Borromean Clinic, or Clinic of the Real (Voruz & Wolf, 2007).[5] What is curious is that after Seminar XI, Lacan will not provide any systematic theorising of anxiety in his teachings. He only mentions it *en passant* once in Seminars XIII and XIV, twice in Seminars XVII and XXII and for the last time in 1977 in his Seminar XXIV, despite the drastic changes to his theories more generally (i.e. the abandonment of the centrality of the Oedipus complex and a detour from a focus on differential diagnosis, both following his move beyond structuralism) (Guéguen, 2013).[6]

[4] Both the Mirror-Stage and the Graph of Desire, which are important graphic representations of Lacan's ideas of the processes of subjectification, the first dating from the late 1940s and the latter from the 1950s and early 1960s, are relevant to an investigation on anxiety. Both concepts deal with the 'mythical' subject that precedes an entry into the Symbolic and early processes of constituting a relation to the Imaginary and the body, therefore implicating the ontology of the Lacanian subject in relation to the negativity of desire. A key text in which this question of subjectification and desire is dealt with is "The Subversion of the Subject and the Dialectic of Desire in the Freudian Unconscious", from 1960, published in *Écrits*.

[5] This matter of a structural lack versus what would be a generative gap or crack is the core of where Lacanian theory can meet Deleuze and Guattari's ideas of the unconscious and desire.

[6] This is significant as moving away from a differential diagnosis, which is based on fixed categories of structural diagnosis (neuroses, psychoses or perversion), accompanies the side-lining of Oedipus in Lacan. Only beyond structural diagnosis and Oedipus that a singularity of the symptom is really being dealt with clinically.

Preliminarily, Lacan holds onto the Freudian idea that anxiety is an affect (Lacan, 1962–1963 [2014], pp. 14, 18) and an 'exceptional affect' (Soler, 2014). For Lacan, it is in anxiety that the Real makes an 'apparition', since "anxiety highlights how much of the subject is not captured by language, or how much is left over after the most exhaustive attempts to encapsulate or represent the subject in words" (Gallagher, 1996, p. 5). It is owing to its relation to the Real that anxiety points at a failure of fantasy, and this is developed in detail through Seminar X, especially in relation to castration anxiety. Fantasy, that for the neurotic structure functions as a cover up for the fundamental 'structural fault', for 'that bit' that is not reflected in the mirror, fails to provide this efficient covering up in the moment of anxiety.[7] This fact alone alludes to something beyond symbolisation, something that fails and in failing is unique to each subject that is evident in anxiety. In addition, we must consider how important it is in the Lacanian orientation, and in psychoanalysis more broadly, to understand anxiety not as an 'isolated symptom', as the dominant discourse within the psy field would have it; rather, it is entangled in psychic experience and fundamental to the treatment.

Anxiety, in this tradition, evidences the *extimate* character of the psychic apparatus. *Extimité* is the Lacanian play on words to emphasise that "the intimate is Other—like a foreign body, a parasite" (Miller, 2008). In this sense, the oft-quoted passage "anxiety is the desire of the Other", which Lacan elaborates in Seminar X, indicates how it is through anxiety that we can 'dig' into the Otherness in oneself and the *self-ness* in the Other. To extrapolate this further, through anxiety we can navigate from an estrangement to a possible entanglement in the I-Other/others relation—this being a possible interpretation of 'vibration'. To arrive there, I will carve the nuances of entanglement in the subject formation proposed by Lacan and alive in clinical practice of this orientation. If anxiety points to a stranger of me as experienced by me, what is the source and extent of such stranger? Is it an abyss-within or a horizon-beyond, as the Freudian articulation from libido, through Oedipus to an Id-perception?

[7] Lacan offers detailed accounts of his concept of fantasy in different moments of his teachings. In general, it describes each subject's specific or unique relation to the object of desire, or *object a*. The most important seminars on the question of fantasy are Seminar IV, *La Relation d'objet* (1956–1957); Seminar VIII, *Le Transfert* (1960–1961) and Seminar *XIV, La Logic du fantasme* (1966–1967).

## Lacan's Mirrors

In 'On Narcissism', from 1914, Freud addresses the constitution of the ego, or what allows the self to become an object in the psychoanalytic sense. However, Freud leaves the question of the 'birth' of such an ego open, simply hinting at a possible 'new psychical action' that must take place in order to allow the 'birth' of the ego, without precisely pointing to what this action would exactly be. Lacan offers an answer to this open-ended question left by Freud with his theory of the Mirror Stage. His inventive response points towards the assimilation of the identification with an external image as what allows for this 'ego' or in general terms a 'self', or an I/Ich, to exist. To Lacan it was partly due to human premature birth—all babies are "trapped in [...] motor impotence and nursling dependence" (Lacan, 1949 [2006], p. 76)—that children are drawn to their reflection in the mirror, a striking image of a 'complete' body, or coherent body in which all limbs and parts of this early '*l'hommelette*' form one's image. This uncanny meeting leads to the identification with a coherent image thereafter; it is, for Lacan, a moment of jubilation. In the first eighteen months of age, for Lacan, the Mirror Stage represents this inaugural encounter with an image of oneself reflected in the mirror, an image which appears, strangely, complete.

As we can trace from his writings of 1949 onwards, the Mirror presents the promise of an image of totality, elaborating psychoanalytic explanations for the dynamics through which the child gravitates towards this image. Since then a certain anticipation for a future mastering of all functions that the child by the time of their encounter with the Mirror does not yet have is present, as is a fictional tone to the identification proposed through the mirror. This 'fiction' of the 'form' (Lacan, 1949 [2006]), as Lacan calls the image, which is constitutive of the subject, comes from an 'outside' space. Or, the m(ego), the subject, reflects back i(a), which is the image from the Other that is constituting this same 'moi'/'ego'. This relation is discussed throughout Seminar I, delivered in 1954. It is, therefore, via the identification with this 'fictional' mirror image that a perception of one's own body comes through. This relation between the body and what Lacan will call the registers of the Imaginary, the Symbolic and the Real will reverberate later on in the Lacanian theories of anxiety.

Preoccupied with the grounds for the emergence of the psychoanalytic subject, Lacan theorises the ego in the manner of a 'return' to Freud that contrasted with a 'mastering' and 'unity' character present in other then dominant schools of psychoanalytic thinking. The image in the mirror appears as a crucial mediator between 'in' and 'out' that troubles a reliance on a 'reality principle'. In summary: "The function of the mirror stage thus turns out, in my view, to be a particular case of the function of imagos, which is to establish a relationship between an organism and its reality—or, as they say, between the *Innenwelt* and the *Umwelt*" (Lacan, 1949 [2006], p. 78). Parting from such images of 'completeness' that the infant does not yet have, as a reference point for a foundational identification, there is an implicated understanding of the ego already relying on the 'outside' rather than in some 'internal' or individualised agency. Identification crosses the image of the body when establishing an 'I', in a relation that is never without conflict, a status guaranteed by the constant dissonance between these realities (internal, external; *Innenwelt, Umwelt*).

The 'orthopaedic' mirror image also reveals the strong bond between libido and the visual that is present in Lacan's text, especially earlier texts and less so in later works, critically observed by feminist scholars such as Jacqueline Rose (1986). 'Reality' and the image are linked in the sense that whenever a child experiences their own subjective 'chaos', they will return to the 'image', or, they will find recourse in the Imaginary. However, this 'unreliability' of the Imaginary, or the mere fact that one could never 'integrate' or 'be' that image in the mirror, makes for its deceptive character. Without stretching our imagination very much, we can see how this proposition challenges the discourses of wellness, for example, since the 'image' is but a fictional promise to cover up psycho-soma 'chaos'.

The Imaginary function of the Mirror is reformulated through the 1950s and 1960s, mostly by offering an emphasis not so much on the power of the image itself but on the presence of an Other, forming a triangle crossing i(a) [the Image in the mirror], m [the moi] and A, the 'big'

Other/Autre. In the early 1950s, in Seminar I, the Symbolic will already make an appearance when Lacan makes a distinction between the Ideal-Ego and the Ego-Ideal in relation to the Mirror Stage. Other teachings from this period such as Seminar II, Seminar V and the paper 'Remarks on Daniel Lagache's Presentation: Psychoanalysis and Personality Structure', from 1960, published as part of the *Écrits*, comment on the fact that in the specular relation there will always be the Other in the equation. Lacan thus swiftly moves beyond the impression of a somewhat 'pure' or 'independent' relation of the infant with the image in the mirror, as described in the 1949 essay, to stress the turn towards the Other. It is crucial to keep in mind that the Lacanian construct of the subject, as a critique of what was then 'mainstream' psychoanalytic theory, marks his efforts to always see any firm reliance on autonomy or an 'individual' crumble. This mark of the Symbolic will be evident in the infant's turn towards the person accompanying them, accessing a confirmatory look from the caring adult that 'glues' the experience of the image on the mirror. In other words, the specular image *i(a)* is constituted via the big Other. The truly "jubilatory" moment in the mirror stage is when the infant turns to the adult: they seem "to be asking the one supporting [them], and here representing the big Other, to ratify the value of this image" (Lacan, 1962–1963 [2014], p. 32).

In sum, from these early 1950s texts, it is clear to us that the Other participates in any specular relation once this experience is not of a 'pure' captivation of the young person by their image. The child's turn towards the Other seeks the recognition that that's 'their image', a Symbolic confirmation ("who is that in the mirror? That is baby", etc.). Already at this stage, Lacan posits the mirror's relation not only to the Imaginary but also to the Symbolic. This is the site of entrance into Lacan's distinctions between the Ego-Ideal and the Ideal-Ego, which are psychic points of reference located in the Symbolic and in the Imaginary registers respectively albeit interconnected. Ideal-Ego is a term that refers to the image in the mirror, the Imaginary point of reference of coherence and completeness that is set into place by the Ego-Ideal, the locus from which the subject feels 'looked at', indexing the site in the Symbolic that frames the subject. Lacan summarised this more complicated Mirror-Schema in the lecture of the 31st of March 1954:

> In other words, it's the symbolic relation which defines the position of the subject as seeing. It is speech, the symbolic relation, which determines the greater or lesser degree of perfection, of completeness, of approximation, of the imaginary. This representation allows us to draw the distinction between the *Idealich* and the *Ichideal*, between the ideal ego and the ego-ideal. The ego-ideal governs the interplay of relations on which all relations with others depend. And on this relation to others depends the more or less satisfying character of the imaginary structuration. (Lacan, 1953–1954 [1991], p. 141)

The Symbolic anchoring of the Ego-Ideal is not arbitrary, or without consequence as Lacan continues:

> The *Ichideal*, the ego-ideal, is the other as speaking, the other in so far as [he] has a symbolic relation to me [moi], which, within the terms of our dynamic manipulation, is both similar to and different from the imaginary libido. Symbolic exchange is what links human beings to each other, that is, it is speech, and it makes it possible to identify the subject. (Lacan, 1953–1954 [1991], p. 142)

The Ego-Ideal is, as it will later be called, the 'unary trait', meaning that it is via the Ego-Ideal that one is able to recognise the other with some trait, or being able to concede that 'this is the Other' through the identification with this unary trait (clearly carrying the tone of universal referential in subjective formation). Lacan will develop this in more detail in Seminar IX on the theme of Identification, claiming that the stability of the Ideal-Ego is granted via the unary trait. Putting it differently, it is in this crossed temporality of registers in which Symbolic identification precedes the mirror that the subject emerges, or in very simple terms, the 'world out there' is already the instance of the Other when we arrive into it. It is only thanks to the Mirror image that the '*moi*' as such emerges, almost as an 'ego' that we dress over our early fragmented body, the *corps morcelé.* The Symbolic, culture and discourse are, thus, integral to the anchor of the subject, who comes into 'being' therein, without many routes into 'becoming' outside of such order.

In short, the simple formula I/S (in which I stands for Imaginary and S for Symbolic) proposes that the image only comes to occupy the space of 'an important image' as such when it relies on the presence of the Symbolic, which situates this image. Registers, throughout Lacanian theory even before the 'knots', which mark his later teachings in the 1970s, are not separate or in blocks, rather, they constantly appeal to each other. This support in the Symbolic was Lacan's first important revision of his theory of the Mirror Stage—a development that is important for his theories on anxiety as we will see in what follows—and allows us to explore the matters of self-consciousness and recognition via the philosophical 'roots' of the Lacanian Mirror.

Self-consciousness as a general philosophical debate that crossed the field of psy in its heart was at the centre of Lacan's reworking of Freudian texts and his own psychoanalytic contributions. With the writings on the Mirror Stage, and subsequent earlier teachings, the centrality of this theme is clear for they condensed fundamental ideas of his thoughts around the installation, development and maintenance of an 'I'. Without running the risk of delineating a metapsychology that favoured adaptation, 'normality' or mastering, Lacan's subject is since the beginning of his teachings marked by a 'glitch' to normality, and concepts such as 'barred', 'alienation', Real, *object a* will offer a side of impossibility, antagonism and excess to any experience of the 'self', both in fantasies as in symptoms (Chiesa, 2007; Van Haute, 2002).

In this sense, the Lacanian praxis elaborates a subjectivity that goes against the grain of the hegemonic psychiatric nosology. Following Freud, the lines between a 'normal' and a 'pathological' are blurred and symptoms, as well as anxiety, appear as lively and dynamic arrangements that each subject finds in order to stay alive. In treatment, mapping the function and modus operandi of such symptoms, as entangled to the body, libido and a general position in the world, is the fundamental logic of its direction. Rather than thinking of a symptom in isolation and 'blocking' it either by avoidance (a process which is integral to CBT techniques, for example) or chemically (with the use of pharmaceutical drugs), exploring how this symptom was formed in the historical narrative of the patient and re-orienting its dynamic to one of less suffering (without any preconceived standard for what that looks like) is what directs the clinic. In Lacan, the barred subject is 'glitched' already, for a coherent 'I' is but an illusion.

## Consciousness and Desire

Already in Lacan's ideas of the Mirror, there is a furthering of the Hegelian dialectic of master and slave as a somewhat stable cycle into a conflict of recognition internal to subjects (yet not restricted to an individual), divided between the 'real me', or my physical perception that is fragmented and incoherent, and 'that me in the mirror', which is really an image of the body of the child, an image of this body in its entirety, with a coherent contour. In simple terms, that reflection on the mirror functions as an 'ideal-I' acting as a point of reference and generates an ongoing impasse between 'reality' and an anchoring 'wholeness or 'coherence' (Lacan, 1949 [2006]). Such coherence will always be deceiving despite being necessary, for what we see in the mirror is an image mediated by the 'external world', by the Symbolic, conferring an essential alienation to subjective experience and removing any possibility of a 'pure' captivation of the subject by the image 'alone'. Hegelian philosophy, through Kojève, influenced Lacan's distrust in the ego as theorised by his contemporaries, mostly Anna Freud, whose work on the ego's defences he is very critical of, since for Lacan the ego should not be seen as "centred on the perception-consciousness system or an organised by the 'reality principle'" (Lacan, 1949 [2006], p. 80). Rather, he argues, we must "take as our point of departure the function of misrecognition that characterises the ego" (Lacan, 1949 [2006], p. 80). An 'impossibility' of sorts in the process of identification will mark the Lacanian subject from then onwards, becoming more evident in his later discussions of the Real. Such 'impossibility', as I am carving out in this book, is the very edge of 'being' and 'becoming' in Lacan.

Crossing 'perception' and 'consciousness', desire is, as various exchanges during his first Seminar show, the fundamental term Lacan takes from philosophy into his psychoanalytic work. In Seminar I, Lacan goes through what he considers to be "the fundamental Hegelian theme—man's desire is the desire of the other" (Lacan, 1953–1954 [1991], p. 146), this being "exactly what is made plain in the model by the plane mirror" (Lacan, 1953–1954 [1991], p. 146). In this Seminar Lacan stresses the relation of 'desire' and the 'other' in the crucial '*moment de virage*', or the 'turning point' in 'development' (and he uses this word here) that is the mirror stage "in which the individual makes a triumphant exercise of his own image in the mirror, of himself" (Lacan, 1953–1954 [1991], p. 146), in which "what occurs here for the first time, is the anticipated seizure of mastery" (Lacan, 1953–1954 [1991], p. 146). This moment is also the first time, he explains when debating with an attendee of his seminar, that one's libido is unstuck, or we could understand that libidinal investments whilst still being narcissistic are detached from the body itself, redirected to the image in the mirror and yet crossing or traversing the 'other', or the Symbolic, and thus producing a delay that evidences a 'gap of desire'. Lacan explicates:

> The subject originally locates and recognises desire through the intermediary, not only of his own image, but of the body of his fellow being. It's exactly at that moment that the human being's consciousness, in the form of consciousness of self, distinguishes itself. It is in so far as he recognises his desire in the body of the other that the exchange takes place. It is in so far as his desire has gone over to the other side that he assimilates himself to the body of the other and recognises himself as body. (Lacan, 1953–1954 [1991], p. 147)

This primordially 'intersubjective' approach to desire, consciousness, perception, relation to one's body and one's image is, as Lacan explains, already present in this version of the Mirror Stage of the 1950s. It is interesting that Lacan spells out the relation between the perception/experience of a fragmented body and a 'fragmented' or not yet 'matured' desire in this pre-Mirror Stage moment of life, explaining that "The body as fragmented desire seeking itself out, and the body as ideal self, are projected on the side of the subject as fragmented body, while it sees the other as perfect body" (Lacan, 1953–1954 [1991], p. 148). Quite confusingly, this very early 'fragmented body' is not 'glued' to the subject, or, it is not 'from the place of the fragmented body' or as an 'I-as-fragmented' that the subject engages with the other and their image. Rather, "for the subject, a fragmented body is an image essentially dismemberable from its body" (Lacan, 1953–1954 [1991], p. 148). What I read from these passages is precisely that subject formation, or the establishment of self-consciousness, in Lacan, is bound to a bodily experience. That is because desire (or a 'singular' mark of being) is 'matured' through the dialectic engagement of the ideal mastery of the body—or of the coherent contour of the body on the mirror—and the body of an other. In this sense, a relation to the world is already 'alienated' from this multiple, fragmented body; channelled through an image captured through its place in culture (an important detail to hold on to, as this fragmented body returns as the central theme of Lacan's later works, after the abandonment of the Oedipal metaphor). Alienation, identification and a certain 'dividualisation' are thus structural to the Lacanian subject, yet, this same theory makes evident the very fictional quality of such identifications, alienations and dividualised subjectivities assumed by psychoanalysis.

In the following sessions, when exploring the 'see-saw' of desire, Lacan will bring into his focus 'identification', making it clear that the establishment of desire is not a simple 'stage' that one goes through once, crossing through the other and the mirror, rather, it is through a series of identifications, a series of encounters, a series of moments of being in the world that desire in its singularity will emerge. Identification, however, is not without a 'problem', since this fundamentally alienated desire should only be 'resolved' with the destruction of the other, as Hegelian dialectics would indicate for Lacan:

> Before desire learns to recognise itself—let us now say the word—through the symbol, it is seen solely in the other. At first, before language, desire exists solely in the single plane of the imaginary relation of the specular stage, projected, alienated in the other. The tension it provokes is then deprived of an outcome. That is to say that it has no other outcome—Hegel teaches us this—than the destruction of the other. The subject's desire can only be confirmed in this relation through a competition, through an absolute rivalry with the other, in view of the object towards which it is directed. And each time we get close, in a given subject, to this primitive alienation, the most radical aggression arises—the desire for the disappearance of the other in so far as he supports the subject's desire. (Lacan, 1953–1954 [1991], p. 170)

This 'destruction of the other' and the question of aggressiveness and this dialectic struggle obviously generate a political matter in Lacan's description of the subject and the possibilities of socialisation. Lacan spells it out simply as "an impossibility of all human coexistence", which I take as a poignant political shortcoming in Lacanianism (or, less generously, a blatant sign of his modern patriarchal and colonial epistemological roots). Yet, he also points that it is via the Symbolic order, or of language, that living together is made possible. In this sense, we are all enigmas to each other that get by through speaking—a relation that carries its limits but that has profound political and clinical implications when considering the relation between the analyst and analysand, the limits of speech and the fitness of diagnosis to the masses under the same names. In Lacanian practice, the enigma of the other and the flimsiness of identification are what prevent the analyst from interpretations (of the transference, of the material brought into the sessions, as done in other clinical orientations) that would be akin to a 'colonisation' of the unconscious, or an act of clinical violence.

The quest for recognition of one's desire in the other is, therefore, the setting stone of the Lacanian psychoanalytic approach and his clinic of a desire that is by essence intersubjective. That means that the subject's desire comes into being through this relation with an other. The Lacanian clinic that aims at unveiling one's desire is fundamentally a clinical approach that situates the subject psychosocially. The Lacanian clinic, it can be argued, is psychosocial *par excellence* once it engages with the fact of the alienation of the I on the image (misrecognition) and in this negativity of desire as a mode of being (Safatle, 2006), and always puts in check the subject and their symptoms as part of a shared matrix rather than an isolated, individual phenomenon. There is a certain level of entanglement in the Lacanian subject, yet, it leaves something behind.

Recognition—or *misrecognition*—of oneself in the image or in the other and the appeal to the Symbolic do not come, however, smoothly or totally. There is always something else involved and it is this that is bound up with the concept of the Real. Anchoring the non-adaptive character of the negativity of desire, the Real already appears in the early writings on the Mirror Stage as embodied in the prematurity of the human child and an early lack of coordination. However, at first, we have 'that' which is there at the beginning—but only mythically—that can be partially subsumed to an image, but not entirely, or this 'me' which does not fit into the image.

Following the logic set out by Lacan with his writings on the Mirror Stage, once identified with the image, the infant starts to gesticulate, to experiment with the space surrounding them, reaffirming that "that is their image" at the same time that "the image is not themselves", opening up, therefore, this other space, a space *outside the mirror*. Whilst the specular image establishes an anchoring point of the subject, it also establishes a space for a 'real' body, its frontiers with the world, a contour. The body, therefore, is essential to identification, from which emerge a complicated relation to the image and, as Lacan adds in early seminars, the Symbolic barring of the subject. From the outset of Lacan's teachings, simply by following the logic delineated in the theory of the Mirror Stage, the body functions as a point of departure to identification at the same time that it never 'fits' into any 'frame' completely. From the body and the experience of being a body or having a body, Lacan will follow Freud in exploring particular bodily parts that in their very 'not-fitting' establish the drives, or as Lacan will call it at the time of Seminar X, the different forms of *object a*. We could say, thus, that this earlier period of Lacan's teachings, during the 1950s, addresses the bodily presence of the subject as an inside out of the mirror from various perspectives. Towards the end of this decade, and moving into the 1960s, this 'in-out' excess, or that of 'me' which cannot fit the cut of the frame of the mirror that appears in the image, becomes more clearly articulated as not only a matter of the Imaginary (or the 'image in the mirror'). Rather, the 'excess' and as its counterpart, 'lack', both on the side of the subject and on the side of the Other, are unravelled in relation to the Symbolic register.

The effect of the Symbolic or, in Lacanian parlance, the effects of the Symbolic 'cut' upon the subject that results precisely in emerging as subject are explored in the 1950s and early 1960s across a variety of teachings, crossing themes that range from identification to transference. In order to offer some clarity on Lacan's articulations in regard to the Real in relation to the Symbolic at this moment of his work, a delineation of his elaboration on 'desire'—which is perhaps the most fundamental concept of Lacanian Psychoanalysis—is of particular relevance. It is in the limits of his theory of desire as harnessed to the desire of the Other and what grounds are then left for the Real that our thinking of anxiety as vibration is articulated.

In Seminar VII, delivered between 1959–1960 on the theme of Ethics of Psychoanalysis, the Real appears, with clarity, as a 'problem of language'. By this is meant that the Real marks what is impossible within language or symbolisation. Lacan delves into the matter of 'impossibility' as a legitimate path to engaging with reality and it is in this respect that the Real as an 'impossibility' is articulated. This seminar, which deals with the relations between action and desire, offers an elaboration of the concept of '*la chose*', *das Ding* or 'the thing', an enigmatic 'excess' that will later form the base of his concept of *object a* as the object cause of desire—crucial contributions of his work on Anxiety. Lacan speaks of a 'field of das Ding' as the locus of an ungraspable enigma that organises psychic life.

In the following year, when teaching about Transference in his Seminar VIII, Lacan returns to the Mirror Stage and the relation between anxiety and desire. Dissecting his formula of fantasy [$ <> a] in relation to Freud's 'Inhibition, Symptom and Anxiety' text, Lacan argues that "anxiety is produced when the cathexis of little *a* is transferred to $" (Lacan, 1960–1961 [2015], p. 361). By this he means that there is something in fantasy that orients the barred S, or the subject, in relation to their desire and this point of apprehension of oneself as desiring is homologous to i(a), the Ideal-Ego, or the Imaginary 'image on the mirror'. Lacan explains that:

> anxiety as a signal is produced somewhere, in a place that can be occupied by i(a)—the ego insofar as it is the image of the other, the ego insofar as it is, fundamentally, the function of misrecognition. It occupies this place not inasmuch as this image occupies it but qua place—in other words, inasmuch as this image can, on occasion, be dissolved there. (Lacan, 1960–1961 [2015], p. 363)

The possibility of this image in the mirror, or the fantasy, or the Imaginary (which are similar to one another, as he points out) being 'dissolved', or 'to fail', brings out anxiety. It is not "the absence of the image that provokes anxiety" (Lacan, 1960–1961 [2015], p. 363), rather it is the encounter with this failure of the fantasy that brings out anxiety. In fact, in Seminar X Lacan will posit that "the structure of anxiety is the structure of the fantasy" (Lacan, 1962–1963 [2014], p. 3). This emergence of anxiety, however, is only possible through a relation to desire, so Lacan's invocation of the order of the fantasy is, in this seminar, simply a way into this relation to one's desire and the same 'way into' can be articulated in regard to the mirror image and the question of the 'object of desire'.

Anxiety does not emerge as facing the image per se, rather, in facing the image as 'a'; or, it is this charge of 'a' present in the specular image and in the fantasy that allow for their function in relation to the emergence of anxiety. He writes: "Anxiety is the radical mode by which a relationship to desire is maintained" (Lacan, 1960–1961 [2015], p. 365). Already in this seminar (VIII) we can sense an anticipation to what Lacan will develop in detail in Seminar X, which is the relation between anxiety and desire through the various forms of the *object a*, granting anxiety the status of the affect that does not 'lie'.

Sustaining one's relation to desire therefore is the function of anxiety. More is elaborated on desire, its emergence and the emergence of the subject, around the same time Lacan was delivering Seminar VIII, in the influential text 'The Subversion of the Subject and the Dialectic of Desire in the Freudian Unconscious', from 1960 and published as part of *Écrits*. In this work, the subject is situated in relation to the establishment of needs, demands and desire, forming an interesting base to what will 'happen' to desire at the moment of Seminar X, a few years later. A concise summary of this article could be as follows: In our attempts to 'satisfy our desire', this desire is transposed by demands, important terms in this analysis of subjectivity. A physical need such as hunger or thirst can be satisfied. However, our 'subjective needs' when transferred to the Other, in the belief this Other could satisfy our desire, take the shape of what Lacan calls a 'demand'. Demands are, in simple terms, a manifestation of desire limited by language, the in-between point, or a gap, in the relation of need and desire (Lacan, 1960 [2006]). The interlinking of desire and the Other demonstrates how the split of the subject also leaves the subject deprived of autonomy, being impossible to gain any sense of selfhood outside of the relationship with culture—'culture', or the Symbolic, is understood by Lacan in a particular and not unproblematic way that is limited to a dialectical relation, where a 'rest' (the Real) can only be accounted as an impossible that is the kernel of symptoms.

At the same time, the body is still present in these elucubrations, being then at the heart of the psychoanalytic project. As Lacan puts it, "psychoanalysis concerns the reality [*réel*] of the body and of its imaginary mental schema" (Lacan, 1960 [2006], p. 680). To illustrate the complex dynamic of subjectivation through desire and the Other, Lacan formulated the Graph of Desire, an evolution of *mathemes* worked across a series of different seminars, noticeably Seminar V and given emphasis in this text and in Seminar X. The basic element of the graph is the '*point de capiton*', a subjective 'point of anchoring' representing the autonomy of the signified and signifier, furthering Saussure's linguistic model of there not being a universal grounding referent for meaning, rather just a structure of signs in relation to one another.[8]

The complete Graph of Desire explores the duality of attempting to gain recognition from the Other in the enterprise of becoming the object of desire of the Other, giving evidence to the *objet a*, the '*petit autre*' in the Imaginary realm. In trying to identify the desire of the Other, the subject identifies with this "what the Other wants from me", a fantasy, attaching the desire of the Other to its own subjective experience (Lacan, 1960 [2006]). From the Graph of Desire, another interesting element of Lacanian thought arises: anxiety. The subjective opacity granted by the prominence of the Other over one's desire leaves a gap, once there is "no universal satisfaction" (Lacan, 1960 [2006], p. 689). This uncertainty, this impossibility, is anxiety. In desire, which opens space for a fantasy of omnipotence of the Other (Lacan, 1960 [2006]), we become subjected to the rules of the Other. Here again, the subject could only gain access to something that could be perhaps called 'oneself' or even 'singularity' not within language, so not within this rule of the Other, but through the repetition of the drive, the force that makes it repeat, or desire, as caused

[8] Guattari moves away from Saussure and Lacan via his study of Glossematics and the linguistic theory proposed by the Danish linguist Hjelmslev, making the relation to meaning and representation more complex in his theory of the unconscious.

by *object a* and opened in something of the order of the rims of the body. These 'rims' have a significant importance when thinking of anxiety beyond the limits of the Oedipus complex. Accordingly, these 'openings' of the body, where in and out get mixed-up or confused, are the loci of the drive; and it is from the logic of the drive, rather than of desire, that Lacan's later teachings get closer to an 'anti-oedipal' model of the unconscious (Schuster, 2016).

## Phallic Troubles

To get to this point, or in order to lay out the ground for a non-Oedipal critique of Lacanian psychoanalysis, it is important that some basic elements of his ideas of the 'phallus', 'lack' and 'sexual difference' are clarified. Once these problematic and widely criticised elements of Lacan's theory appear with evidence in his work on anxiety as well. We can start from the premise, as seen above, that negotiating one's 'reality' with the idealised version of oneself through discourse leaves behind an excess, an 'un-symbolisable' fragment, the Real (as described in his early teachings and in relation to the Imaginary). Subjects will be left in a constant "discordance with [their] own reality" (Lacan, 1949, p. 2) in the same manner that the positioning of oneself in language will leave out a frustrating lack (again, the Real comes in his mid-life teachings as a 'gap' in the Symbolic system). Desire will carry in its core an absence, a lack. The unconscious, therefore for Lacan, is marked by lack, one we will try to fulfil throughout life with no necessary guarantee of success. The understanding that desire will never be satiated, that one's wish for wholeness will always be frustrated, is the meaning Lacan attached to the phallus (Lacan, 1958). As a 'veiled signifier', the phallus marks the divide inherent to subjectivity. It is that which guarantees the Imaginary with Symbolic 'support', with a promise in language. Symbolising, thus, brings reassurance. This use of the word 'phallus' and further developments of theories of femininity leave space for pertinent feminist critiques (Braidotti, 1994).

The Mirror Stage can be utilised as a fruitful background for thinking of the split subject, one of Lacan's greatest contributions to the thinking of subjectivity. Whilst the divide of the subject already refutes any notion of unity, Lacan proposes femininity and masculinity 'lack differently'. The 'Law of the Father', which guarantees prominence to the phallus in culture, can be understood as Lacan's denunciation of patriarchy (Mitchell, 1982; Rose, 1986). When theorising on sexual difference—in *Encore* Lacan, curiously, does not cite any women analyst—and positing that '*Woman does not exist*', Lacan denounces biological roles as determinant, yet, he backs this idea by stipulating different 'kinds' of *jouissance* experienced by 'men' and 'women' (in Seminar XX—Lacan, 1972–1973). Phallic jouissance is the frustrating enjoyment in believing we have satiated our desire, a promise held in the Other; whilst the 'Other jouissance' involves carrying this 'promise' of satisfaction in oneself. The Lacanian views of sexual difference and the phallus will then move from a strict guarantor of lack, which flirts with biologism in the 1958 text 'The Signification of the Phallus', which was published in *Écrits,* to his first views of 'different' kinds of jouissance in Seminar X on Anxiety (when he still speaks of the breast, breastfeeding and the detumescence of the phallus/penis) until the clear formulation of sexual difference in Seminar XX, where a 'masculine' and a 'feminine' position are the (only, for him) two options of a relation to the phallic Law that mark two different subject positions. This Law comes in as a mediator of the 'excessive' jouissance, in which 'everyone lacks', but just 'enjoy' differently. 'Lack' is throughout Lacan's teachings an anchor of subject formation, one that presents in 'negativity' its antidote beyond total domination. The deep interconnection of these themes in Lacanian teachings makes it very difficult for some theorists and psychoanalysts to try and conceive of a subjectivity that is not dependent upon Oedipal sexual difference (and its binary arrangement) or on 'lack'. Addressing the political and onto-epistemic problems of this far from neutral arrangement that relies on the binary of sexual difference seems to cause a crisis of imagination among orthodox followers of Lacanian texts. Owing to this, tensions between feminist theory and psychoanalysis seem to be as alive as ever, with a current of Lacanian analysts equating, for example, transgender living to psychosis precisely on the grounds of such 'lack' being foreclosed.

Contemporary elaborations around queerness and trans-identities in psychoanalytic settings have argued that transgender subjectivity sits on the side of psychosis (Millot, 1990; Morel, 2000). That would be because it is a case of foreclosure of the Name-of-the-Father and a push-to-the-woman (inspired by the reading of Schreber's case) characteristic of the inability to live with the inconsistency of sexuality, transitioning thus as a way to name oneself and suture this gap.[9] Argentinean analyst Patricia Gherovici (2017), however, has led the way in stating what, to me at least, is the obvious reality of the Lacanian psychoanalytic encounter: trans people, like all people, can have any unconscious structure and can be hysterics just as well. Whilst Gherovici's (2017) remarks are well grounded in case-studies and theory and her contributions are generous and therapeutically sound, there is still some insistence on the equation of sexual difference (and differential diagnoses) as fundamental to the clinical encounter and to subjective formation. What Gherovici does is very important: as a clinician and keen theorist of Lacan's teachings, she finds a ground within Lacanian theory to demonstrate how queerness can be a creative solution of a capacity to live without the hold of the phallus. In other words, rather than a symptomatic escape, it is a *sinthôme*, like James Joyce's *sinthôme*—described in Lacan's seminar XXIII, from 1975–1976.[10] By acknowledging a possibility that is not 'just' psychosis

[9] Miller (2021), following this very logic, has generated much negative response to his 'Docile au Trans' article in response to Preciado's (2020) intervention at the École de la cause Freudienne de Paris in 2019, such is the difficulty of the Lacanian field in abandoning sexual difference as its core onto-epistemic pillar.

[10] Lacan says, in Seminar XXIII, in the lesson of the 18th of November 1975: "Joyce expresses himself as one might expect from him in a very pertinent way. I mean that he metaphorises something which is nothing less than his relationship to his body. He notes that the whole affair has drained away. He expresses this by saying that it is like a fruit skin. What does this indicate to us? This indicates to us that this something that is already so imperfect in all human beings, the relationship to the body—who knows what is happening in his body? It is clear that there is here indeed something which is extraordinarily suggestive and which, even for some, is the meaning they give, it is certain, these people in question, it is the meaning they give to the Unconscious. But there is something that I, from the beginning, have articulated with care, which is precisely the fact that the Unconscious, has nothing to do with the fact that one is ignorant of a lot of things concerning one's own body. And that what one knows is of a quite different nature. One knows things that that have to do with the signifier; the old notion of the Unconscious, of the *Unbekannte,* was precisely something based on our ignorance of what is happening in our bodies. But Freud's Unconscious, is something that is worthwhile stating on this occasion, it is precisely what I said. Namely, the relationship, the relationship between a body which is foreign to us which is a circle, indeed an infinite straight line, which in any case are one and the other equivalent, and something which is the Unconscious. So then what meaning are we to give to what Joyce bears witness to? Namely, that it is not simply the relationship to his body. It is, as I might say, the psychology of this relationship which... for after all, psychology is nothing other than that, namely, this confused image we have of our own body, but this confused image does not fail to include, let us call them what they are called, affects".

to whatever mode of existing that does not correspond to the phallic Law, Gherovici paves the way for a feminist conceptualisation of all forms of rupture with 'the phallus' as creative transformation within the *sinthôme*.[11] Accordingly, and informing my theory of anxiety as vibration, excess, chaos or too-muchness (such as anxiety) do not necessarily need to be 'castrated' in order to be soothed—as Gherovici (2018) herself proposed elsewhere—nor 'sublimated', rather, excess can be mobilised into a *sinthôme*, bypassing the Law-of-the-Father into a 'becoming'. This possibility, or, what is done to 'excess' is central to Lacan's seminar on anxiety.

## Seminar X: L'Angoisse

When Lacan started his Seminar on Anxiety (Seminar X, in 1962–1963) the first lectures brought up again the Mirror Stage and the Graph of Desire, demonstrating how the Other is inscribed in the specular relation. To Lacan, anxiety was an affect separating desire and *jouissance* (Harari, 2001) in which the fear of fragmentation is paramount. Reworking Freud's earlier ideas of an anxiety which anticipates a threat to the ego, Lacan points anxiety towards the Imaginary. The virtual specular image and its prestigious state attract the subject. The subject invests more and more in their own body—believed to be the originator of the specular image—with the aid of objects assuming the role of the object of desire; being, consequently, fooled (Lacan, 1962–1963). This dynamic precisely was named 'anxiety' at the lecture of November 28, 1962. The 'strange' object that Lacan discovers, *object a*, is the focus of several of the lessons of the seminar on anxiety, once "anxiety is not incited by the lack of the object but rather by the lack of the lack, i.e. the emergence of an object in the place of lack" (Salecl, 2004, p. 32), standing right in between desire and *jouissance*. Once desire is linked to frustration and the lack of

[11] *Sinthôme* is a term Lacan introduces in 1975 as a rewriting of the symptom. As a singular manner of enjoyment that does not call for interpretation, resting beyond the Symbolic, the *sinthôme* (a play on the words 'saint' and 'man', in French), appears as a fourth element of the Borromean knot, tying imaginary, Symbolic and Real together. In Seminar XXIII, *Le Sinthôme*, it appears as creative solution in the organisation of libido/enjoyment or *jouissance* that makes no use of the Imaginary; or a creative solution to carry on living.

the object of satisfaction, *jouissance* is the somewhat 'painful'—or 'charged'—approach to this satisfaction; enjoyment, or the Lacanian version of Freud's libido. The 'lack of lack', the knowledge something is there which could satisfy our desire and yet, it does not, appearing in the place where lack should be, is in this complicated logic, the backbone of anxiety. The new argument brought forward by Lacan in this seminar is the fact that there will always be a portion of the libido that does not go through the Mirror image (elaborated in terms of the *minus phi,* castration and *object a*). The image in this seminar is defined by the exclusion of *minus phi* and *object a*, leaving something aside. If the 'lack lacks', it then produces the affect of anxiety. An auto-erotic *jouissance*, something that is profoundly invested in the body makes its way in anxiety; in other words, in anxiety, the Symbolic is invaded by the Real and desire appears as extracted, indexed to the experience that we are only just bodies (hence the bodily harnessing and mobilisation of anxiety, both in a chronic form and in attacks).

Anxiety is an "intermediary term between jouissance and desire in so far as desire is constituted and founded upon the anxiety phase, once anxiety has been got through" (Lacan, 1962–1963 [2014], p. 175), writes Lacan in an often-quoted passage from Seminar X. What is very important in this seminar is the idea of 'going through' anxiety. In French, the original term used is '*franchir*', thus '*franchir l'angoisse*' connotes a stepping through it as if stepping over a threshold, crossing it. Lacan is referring to castration anxiety, saying that only when one crosses through one's castration anxiety can desire be encountered. This idea presents an interesting paradox, bringing up a cyclical impossibility of our relation both to anxiety and desire. We could parallel here an idea from Lacan's Seminar VII, of '*ceder*', or giving up of one's desire; he states that "from an analytical point of view, the only thing of which one can be guilty is of having given ground relative to one's desire" (Lacan, 1959–1960 [1997], p. 319). In this sense, whenever one goes in the direction of one's desire one feels anxious—as anxiety is a way into desire, as per Seminar VIII—conversely, when one 'gives up' on desire there comes guilt. This is an interesting nuance that is added to the 'truth' found in anxiety in Seminar X. In this sense, there is no 'cure' for anxiety other than desire. The paradox is that in order to access desire you face anxiety, and as a 'cure' to anxiety, there is only desire. There is a cycle here and perhaps the whole notion of '*franchir l'angoisse*' or crossing through one's anxiety that is so central to Lacan's presentation in this seminar implicates a learning to balance oneself within this cycle, or to dance in this rhythm established by anxiety and desire that, as we cannot lose sight of, emerges in the encounter with the Real via the sight of the *object a*.

There is something about anxiety, which is an affect, that is revealing of the structure of the subject, in Lacan's words: "What is anxiety? We've ruled out the idea that it might be an emotion. To introduce it, I will say that it's an affect" (Lacan, 1962–1963 [2014], p. 14). He continues: "And this is even the reason why it has a close structural relationship to what a subject is. On the other hand, what I said about affect is that it isn't repressed. Freud says it just as I do. It's unfastened, it drifts about. It can be found displaced, maddened, inverted, or metabolised. But it isn't repressed. What are repressed are the signifiers that moor it" (Lacan, 1962–1963 [2014], p. 14). Anxiety is, therefore, "a question of desire" (Lacan, 1962–1963 [2014], p. 15). It is owing to such a privileged presence in psychic life that Lacan dedicates a whole year of his teachings to anxiety. A guiding thread into reading this Seminar will be formulated in what follows. It is by carefully looking into Lacan's only major work on the topic of anxiety in detail that an important impasse (or even contradiction in his work) can be fleshed out, namely, how the object of anxiety—*object a*—is not bound to the field of the Other and to the Symbolic, potentially escaping an Oedipal binary of sexual difference frame for the subject.

The Seminar begins with Lacan recuperating Freud's account of anxiety, which is mainly castration anxiety according to his reading of 'Inhibition, Symptom and Anxiety', by means of a theoretical reconstruction. Lacan approached castration anxiety from the point of the dominance of the Symbolic order over the Imaginary, when the latter is then bound to the Symbolic rule. He comments in the first chapters that his contribution in this seminar will be to formulate an anxiety that is 'beyond' castration anxiety. By that he means that everything of the order of the signifier (with a chapter title announcing this precisely: *Anxiety in the Net of Signifiers*) is a castration anxiety. A critical idea that marks Lacan's development of anxiety at the moment of Seminars X and XI is that anxiety is tied with the desire of the Other. Therefore, to address this point, Lacan makes use of the Graph of desire, proposing "a formula indicating the essential relationship between anxiety and the desire of the Other" (Lacan, 1962–1963 [2014], p. 5), stressing that what he added in the then recent work was precisely the matter of the 'desire of the Other'. It is through the elaboration of the desire of the Other that Lacan is able to advance on Freud's theories of castration anxiety. The question '*Che vuoi*?' at the top of the Graph is, thus, an anguishing question. Lacan says "'*Che vuoi*?' is not just 'what does the Other want with me?', it's 'what does [He] want concerning the place of the ego?'" (Lacan, 1962–1963 [2014], p. 6). In other words, this question is linked to the specular image and to narcissistic capture. In the Graph of Desire, "the distance between [the two levels] renders the relationship to desire at once homologous with and distinct from narcissistic identification" (Lacan, 1962–1963 [2014], p. 6). Anxiety, as he points out, plays a role in "the dialectic that knots these two levels [of the Graph] so tightly together" (Lacan, 1962–1963 [2014], p. 6).

Lacan also recuperates ideas from Seminars VIII and IX in relation to the object and the desire of the Other, elucidating an anxiety that is beyond castration anxiety, which is the anxiety facing the desire of the Other, when one is the object for the Other. An anxiety, thus, knitted within the Symbolic realm. Lacan's dissection of the Symbolic, Desire of the Other and Anxiety is rather extensive as he addresses philosophical texts (Hegel and Kierkegaard, especially) and composes multiple formulas to trace what this relation is in the moment of anxiety. This is Lacan's 'structural' approach, where he is looking for the function of the signifier in anxiety in order to trace a map towards the point of anxiety that is beyond the signifier, or how do we cope with the 'rest' in the process of subjectivation.

The 'rest' is very important to the argument that will follow in regard to anxiety and the Real, an articulation that will carry on in the later 1970s with Lacan's last teachings. The rest raises a question of what is left from our *jouissance* when we enter the Other and the field of the signifier. At this point, in Seminar X, he brings us the concept of the 'unary trait'—which stands in very simple words for the fact that there's no subject without a signifier preceding it. In Lacan's words: "There's no conceivable advent of a subject as such except on the basis of the prior introduction of a signifier, and the most straightforward of signifiers, known as the unary trait" (Lacan, 1962–1963 [2014], p. 21). This 'dominance' of the Symbolic is very clear at this point. "The unary trait precedes the subject" (Lacan, 1962–1963 [2014], p. 21) and brings with it a singularity, which he proposes as the "singularity of the trait, this is what we cause to enter the real, whether the real likes or not" (Lacan, 1962–1963 [2014], p. 21). This unary trait marks the subject in the sense that it mediates the speaking subject's access to the Real whilst it is, itself, extracted from the field of the Other, which, in its turn, precedes the subject. This articulation reads slightly confusingly, but one simple manner to connect it with anxiety is the following: once the subject is marked with the unary trait, drawn from the field of the Other, a relation to the Other is instigated that moves the subject towards an encounter with the Other's desire. Clearly, Lacan leaves very little space for real social emancipation, change or rupture, once the subject seems to be caught by a dominant Symbolic. In other words, there is 'being', but virtually no 'becoming'.

By means of the unary trait, the subject is "inscribed as a quotient" of (i.e. the result of mathematical operation of division by) the Other. In Lacan's words, "first off, you find A, the originative Other as locus of the signifier, and S, the subject as yet inexistent, who has to situate himself as determined by the signifier" (Lacan, 1962–1963 [2014], p. 26). What follows is a move into the Imaginary in relation to anxiety, which is explored by Lacan via Freud's work on narcissism and the Mirror Stage, and it is in this relation that Lacan points to the 'object of anxiety'. Here the concept of the phallus is utilised in order to approach this 'special' object—'special' because Freud had postulated that anxiety had no object and Lacan will 'discover' or reveal the object of anxiety. The phallus, according to his logic, not having an image in the mirror, which is akin to the Imaginary definition of castration, leaves a gap, a void, and it in the space of this lack that something else can appear, in Lacan's words: "the disruption wherein anxiety is evinced arises when this void is totally filled in" (Lacan, 1962–1963 [2014], p. 65). The phallus is auto-erotically invested, giving rise to a fracture in the specular image, this fracture in the specular image is the 'support' of symbolic castration. This 'something else' that can appear in this space is precisely the object of anxiety. The limits to the specular investment are articulated not only through what is left or what remains—Lacan is clear that "not all of the libidinal investment passes by way of the specular image. There's a remainder" (Lacan, 1962–1963 [2014], p. 38)—but also through what is just 'not there'. The remainder is the place of the phallus, which is "an operative reserve" but is "not represented at the level of the imaginary" and is "cut out of the specular image" (Lacan, 1962–1963 [2014], p. 38). This cut can establish two different pieces, first a piece which can have a specular image, which is the *minus phi* and, second, a piece that doesn't have a specular image which is the *object a*.

Lacan underlines the difficulty of defining *object a*, so perhaps the easier manner to grasp it, at least within this seminar is by considering that "whenever Freud speaks of the object of anxiety, think of him as speaking of the object a" (Lacan, 1962–1963 [2014], p. 40). To map the relation between the phallus, *minus phi* and the *object a*, Lacan brings back the mirror stage, positing, in this way that castration anxiety is Imaginary in the sense that "in everything that concerns taking one's bearings in the imaginary, the phallus will henceforth step in, in the form of a lack" (Lacan, 1962–1963 [2014], pp. 39–40). Pointing at the Imaginary, or the image of the body in the mirror, Lacan describes the phallus as essentially 'cut out' of the image, which is why in this seminar the phallus is still considered one of the forms of the *object a*.

Minus-phi, in its turn, denotes the place of such a missing or lacking imaginary phallus. The phallus "can't be grasped in the imaginary", rather it is an absence that brings with it the possibility of presence (Lacan, 1962–1963 [2014], p. 45). Lacan links it strongly to the penis in this seminar with all the references to the body, detumescence and copulation, opening, of course, space for a feminist critique of his view of the phallic function and the predominance of the visual in the Imaginary (and proof that the use of the word phallus is not at all arbitrary but intentional in his work). The phallus as this ungraspable part of the body schema in the Imaginary means, for Lacan, the portion of auto-erotic enjoyment that the subject has not parted with under the castration threat. If minus-phi holds out the possibility of the missing something becoming present in the specular image, the *object a* is a remainder that cannot be brought into the specular field. A relationship is established between this place of lack and the 'libidinal reserve', which could not be incorporated into the specular image and remains profoundly invested at the level of one's body. Lacan calls it primary narcissism, autoeroticism and "an autistic jouissance".

A proximity of the object is the core of Lacan's view on anxiety at this stage of his work. Anxiety, as he stresses time and time again in this seminar, is not without object, neither a signal of lack, but rather it is when the support that this very lack or gap provides to the subject fails that anxiety emerges. Lacan speaks of the baby's relation to the breast, this early encounter with the field of the Other and with the object of anxiety, stressing that is not an anticipation for the breast that produces anxiety, but the anticipation of its going away. He says: "Don't you know that it's not longing for the maternal breast that provokes anxiety, but its imminence? What provokes anxiety is everything that announces to us, that lets us glimpse, that we're going to be taken back onto the lap" (Lacan, 1962–1963 [2014], p. 53). This early encounter is anxiety-provoking once it disrupts the delineation of desire that is then orienting the subject:

> The most anguishing thing for the infant is precisely the moment when the relationship upon which he's established himself, of the lack that turns him into desire, is disrupted, and this relationship is most disrupted when there's no possibility of any lack, when the mother is on his back all the while, and especially when she's wiping his backside. (Lacan, 1962–1963 [2014, pp. 52–3)

The mother being there which is bound to her not being there is what opens space for this anxiety, as he points out. In general terms, anxiety is then not linked to a 'loss' but with a 'presence'. In Lacan's words, "anxiety isn't about the loss of the object, but its presence" (Lacan, 1962–1963 [2014], p. 53). In this sense, and referring back to his work on the seminars on Transference and Fantasy, it is the meeting of a fantasy over the mirror that allows for an object to appear in this space of a void, and when this happens, anxiety emerges. This is what is meant by the often-quoted definition of anxiety being 'the lack of the lack', or, instead of this void, the object pops up. Lacan claims to have discovered such an object, which was only possible after he revised Freud's work in light of his own return to Freud and theoretical advances.

When approaching this object in order to delineate anxiety, Lacan goes through the question of the drive. At the point of Seminar X, the relation between drive and body is on the basis of the action of the signifier over the body. Lacan is also critical of the psychological and psychoanalytic methods to research and theorise anxiety that take as a given that the body is a unity—and here we sense again a strong presence of his earlier critique of phenomenology too. His body is one of excesses. The place of the void and a 'residue' will bring us back to his earlier texts on the Mirror Stage when asking how does the drive is established, or how does the drive 'come about'. Here it is clear that the drive derives from the relation to the mirror image that 'cuts into' the body. The initial *corps morcele*, the fragmented body is cut through when reflected in the mirror and as a result various 'parts' of the body are cut off, or become objects. This cut, therefore, creates lost objects and 'voids' in the body as a graphic ground in which to explore this question of 'these voids' that are established through the cut:

> It is *with* the real image, constituted, when it emerges, as *i(a)* that one clasps or not the multiplicity of objects *a,* here represented by the real flowers, in the neck of the vase, and this is thanks to the concave mirror at the far end, a symbol of something that must stand to be found in the structure of the cortex, the foundation of a certain relationship that man has with the image of his body, and with the different objects that can be constituted from this body, with the fragments of the original body grasped or not at the moment when *i(a)* has the opportunity of being constituted. (Lacan, 1962–1963 [2014], p. 118)

These peculiar, special objects marked on the body are not external, but neither are they completely internal. Such 'inside-out' zigzagging is of the order of the *ex-timate*, of that which is internal but always crossed by the field of the Other. With the *object a* marking such excess of the body that is not captured by the division and establishment of the body and the drives, Lacan comes close to the polymorphous perversion of early Freud and of the Body-Without-Organs of Deleuze and Guattari. For

Lacan, however, and crucially, without the cut, there is no subject. Or, in Lacan's view, there is simply no subject before the mirror stage and whatever there is there, involved in the autoerotic jouissance is not the subject. In his words:

> Prior to the mirror stage, that which will be i(a) lies in the disorder of the objects *a* in the plural and it is not yet a question of having them or not. This is the true meaning, the deepest meaning, to be given to the term *autoeroticism*—one lacks any self, as it were, completely and utterly. It is not the outside world that one lacks, as it is quite wrongly expressed, it is oneself. (Lacan, 1962–1963 [2014], pp. 118–119)

The voids of the body, or the 'rims', as in these physical spaces where in-out get blurred (openings such as the mouth, the anus, the eye, etc.) are loci of the drive only in so far as they bear a relation to the field of the Other, producing an excess that is cast off from this Other. As Lacan puts it: "Freud tells us that anxiety is a rim phenomenon, a signal that is produced at the ego's limit when it is threatened by something that must not appear. This is the *a,* the remainder, which is abhorred by the Other" (Lacan, 1962–1963 [2014], p. 119). The *object a*, therefore, escapes the Symbolic and in this way, causes anxiety, as "if what is seen in the mirror is anguishing, it is in so far as it cannot be proposed to the Other's acknowledgement" (Lacan, 1962–1963 [2014], p. 120). In this sense, anxiety, as an encounter with the Real, is excessive of the field of the Other. By being so, it is excessive to the Oedipal logic and bears a special place within a Lacanian differential diagnosis.

By conducting this very close reading of this seminar, we are able to identify a subtle and yet powerful change to his structural clinic: If psychosis, neurosis and perversion relate to a foreclosure or internalisation of the Name-of-the-Father (Oedipal order), anxiety is an affect that brings the subject to the world beyond such subjective formation: it is a new horizon of being. This is precisely what 'becoming' entails. If anxiety, thus, is an affect that characterises the emergence of experience beyond 'the subject', it moves away from 'being' into a 'becoming'—anxiety vibrates in its emergence. Here is the impasse of Lacan's seminar on anxiety that such close reading allows us to observe.

## Anxiety in Late Lacan

The ethics of Lacanian Psychoanalysis through the relation to Desire and the Real changes in his later teachings. In 'early' Lacan, and in particular in Seminar VII, the seminar dedicated to the *Ethics of Psychoanalysis*, Lacan proposes a version of 'ethics' that can be roughly summarised as an unconditional fidelity to one's singular desire. A simple critique of this notion is that in social life (i.e. collective, political and even democratic life) this arrangement would be 'impossible', for how could we 'fit' in so many singularities, making concessions and negotiations of desire the crux of sociality and subjectivity? In Lacan's later teachings, he offers a second proposition of an ethics of psychoanalysis; without annihilating this principle of fidelity to one's desire, he proposes another ethics that has to do with the Real. He proposed that we must make ourselves 'dupes' of the Real, demarcating thus the later Lacanian characteristic of an 'Ethics of the Real'. Dupe derives from Lacan's poetic linguistic games that take the 'Nom-du-Pere' and 'Pere-version' to the fore, arriving at a 'dupe' of 'du-Pere'. If anxiety is so closely linked to the Real, how does this later ethical proposition relate to anxiety?

The theoretical and clinical potency of anxiety we find in Seminar X was last evoked by Lacan in Seminar XI, when he defends that the clinician must 'canalise' it in 'small doses' in the treatment. Any later mentions of anxiety (the French *angoisse*) will not cover any further theoretical grounds. His very last definition of anxiety comes in 1977, in Seminar XXIV, *L'Insu que Sait de L'Une-Bévue S'Aile à Mourre* (1976–1977), where he characterises anxiety as '*symboliquement réel*' and the opposite of a 'lie'. Until Seminar XI, Lacan delineates an anxiety in relation to the Other and introduces this affect to this peculiar excessive blind-spot he calls *object a*. Towards his later works, we find a change from the structuralist Lacan of desire into a post-structuralist Lacan of the Drive, or of the body, of *jouissance* not harnessed to the Other and beyond the logic of the signifier.

In the 1974 Rome congress of the EFP, Lacan, in what is known as *La Troisième*, says that anxiety is "precisely something that is situated in our body but in another part, it is the feeling that emerges of this suspicion which fools us that we are reduced to our bodies" (Lacan, 1974, p. 102).[12] Around this period, Lacan was reworking fundamental pillars of his teachings such as castration and sexual difference, leaving behind the 'feminine' and 'phallic' *jouissance* he still hung on to in the 1960s. By the time Lacan delivers Seminar XX, in 1972–1973, instead of a phallic *jouissance* (limited by castration) versus the 'other' *jouissance* (beyond castration and object loss), Lacan proposes that it is the signifier that is the main source of *jouissance*. The signifier here appears with a very different face; rather than attached to the possibilities of meaning which dressed his structuralist tone until the 1960s, now the signifier is quite material, it is not bound to meaning but rather to sounds that mark the body in *lalangue* (the lallation of a baby's play with sounds, repetitions and the body, our first encounter with words that will only later be restricted to meaning). Whilst the later Lacan focuses on the *parlêtre*—or the speaking-being—rather than the subject of Oedipal sexual difference, offering a queer possibility for a psychoanalytic subject not determined by the phallic signifier, it is the Real that marks his clinical and theoretical shift.

Voruz and Wolf, two contemporary Lacanian analysts, stress the insistence of the Real as a motor to psychoanalytic theory observable in the transformations of both Freudian and Lacanian texts and seminars through their lifetime (Voruz & Wolf, 2007). Whilst Freud leaves us with the somewhat generalised idea of 'negative therapeutic reactions', Lacan, "eventually had to acknowledge the impossibility of fully 'draining' the unconscious with the signifier" (Voruz & Wolf, 2007, p. viii) and the end of analysis and of his theoretical endeavour. This 'push-to-the-Real', or this unconscious beyond what can be grasped or reduced is, for the psychoanalysts, the characteristic of Lacan's later teachings. Anxiety, and the seminar on anxiety, roughly situated in the middle of Lacan's career and right before his excommunication from the IPA, is, as we know, an encounter with the Real.

Both in Seminar XXII and in *La Troisième,* Lacan puts anxiety in the centre of his Borromean Knot (a diagram of the Imaginary, Symbolic and

[12] My translation from Valas Spanish text (the original printed version of this speech). In Spanish: "*La angustia es, precisamente, algo que se situa en nuestro cuerpo en otra parte, es el sentimiento que surge de esa sospecha que nos embarga de que nos reducimos a nuestro cuerpo*" (Lacan, 1974, p. 102).

Real and its intersections). In this movement, as Colette Soler (2014) also concludes, we are then able to find an anxiety that lies outside meaning, but not outside of the body. This later Lacanian understanding of the Real, which is not an impossibility of the Symbolic but existing outside of it, will not manifest itself as enjoyed meaning (*sens-joui*), rather, it will manifest in the affect of anxiety. Thus, anxiety is an encounter with a materiality of the body that does not cross meaning or the Symbolic (and its discontents). Anxiety can, in this manner, point towards the constitution of a new Imaginary—rather than an abyss within, a whole new horizon. This new horizon takes anxiety as being a 'compass' (Miller, 2007) to the clinic not only of 'being' but also of 'becomings'. In this sense, anxiety is an affect that vibrates possibilities within and beyond the frame of the subject.

A lot has been written in recent years about later Lacanian teachings, a large part of which remains untranslated into English. Lacan, who died in 1981, had a chance to circulate around very radical and political thinkers of his time, from Guattari and Deleuze to the strong feminist movement in France, choosing, however, not to engage so actively with more radical ideas (Dosse, 2010). Aside from a clue to his own political conservativeness, open dialogues between Lacanian works and both feminist and Deleuze and Guattari-influenced thinking have been articulated in academia ever since. However, the lack of a substantial later formulation of anxiety by Lacan could be the reason why anxiety rarely, if ever, features as part of such novel dialogues.

This chapter has mapped Lacan's theory of anxiety whilst articulating it with the potential openings from 'being' into 'becoming' found in his Seminar X. By situating his only systematic theory of anxiety contextually and in detail within Lacan's praxis, it is possible to grasp precisely how the moment of anxiety—in theory, in the clinic and in the experience of this affect—is witness to the emergence of the Real. The Real in question, following this detailed account of his seminars, appears in Seminar X, as still laced by the limits of the Other. The fragmented, or multiple body that Lacan addresses very early on (in Seminars I and II), returns in his later teachings as giving rise to the speaking-body; or the affective body which is not reliant on the Symbolic (and its Oedipal myth). Lacan, however, does not spell out a new theory of anxiety in the

1970s and it is here, recuperating the two vibrational moments in Freud's work on anxiety (namely, the pre-psychoanalytic libidinal excess and the very late Id-excess), that I situate my psychosocial theory of anxiety.

## References


Braidotti, R. (1994). *Nomadic Subjects: Embodiment and Sexual Difference in Contemporary Feminist Theory*. Columbia University Press.

Chiesa, L. (2007). *Subjectivity and Otherness. A Philosophical Reading of Lacan*. The MIT Press.

Dosse, F. (2010). *Gilles Deleuze & Félix Guattari: Intersecting Lives*. Columbia University Press.

Freud, S. (1914). On Narcissism. In *The Standard Edition of the Complete Psychological Works of Sigmund Freud, Volume XIV (1914–1916): On the History of the Psycho-Analytic Movement, Papers on Metapsychology and Other Works* (pp. 67–102). The Hogarth Press and the Institute of Psychoanalysis.

Gallagher, C. (1996). High Anxiety—A Theoretical and Clinical Challenge to Psychoanalysis. *The Letter., 06*(Spring), 1–23.

Gherovici, P. (2017). *Transgender Psychoanalysis: A Lacanian Perspective on Sexual Difference*. Routledge.

Gherovici, P. (2018). Anxious? Castration is the Solution! *Psychoanalytic Inquiry., 38*(1), 83–90.

Guéguen, P.-G. (2013). Who Is Mad and Who Is Not? On Differential Diagnosis in Psychoanalysis. *Culture/Clinic, 1*, 66–85.

Harari, R. (2001). *Lacan's Seminar 'On Anxiety' An Introduction*. Other Press.

Lacan, J. (1945). Logical Time and the Assertion of Anticipated Certainty. In *Écrits:* The First 'Complete Edition in English (2006) [B. Fink, Trans.]. W.W. Norton and Company.

Lacan, J. (1949). The Mirror Stage as Formative of the I Function as Revealed in Psychoanalytic Experience. In *Écrits:* The First 'Complete Edition in English (2006) [B. Fink, Trans.]. W.W. Norton and Company

Lacan, J. (1953). The Function and Field of Speech and Language in Psychoanalysis. In *Écrits:* The First 'Complete Edition in English (2006) [B. Fink, Trans.]. W.W. Norton and Company

Lacan, J. (1957). The Instance of the Letter in the Unconscious, or Reason Since Freud. In *Écrits:* The First Complete Edition in English (2006) [B. Fink, Trans.]. W.W. Norton and Company

Lacan, J. (1958). The Signification of the Phallus. In *Écrits:* The First Complete Edition in English (2006) [B. Fink, Trans.]. W.W. Norton and Company
Lacan, J. (1960). The Subversion of the Subject and the Dialectic of Desire in the Freudian Unconscious. In *Écrits:* The First Complete Edition in English (2006) [B. Fink, Trans.]. W.W. Norton and Company
Lacan, J. (1964). Position of the Unconscious. In *Écrits:* The First Complete Edition in English (2006) [B. Fink, Trans.]. W.W. Norton and Company
Lacan, J. (1966). *Écrits*. Les Éditions du Seuil.
Lacan, J. (1974). *La Tercera.* [Online]. https://www.valas.fr/IMG/pdf/JLACAN_La_tercera.pdf
Lacan, J. (1975). *Seminar XXIII,* Lesson of the 18th of November, 1975. Gallagher's translation. [Online]. http://www.lacaninireland.com/web/wp-content/uploads/2010/06/THE-SEMINAR-OF-JACQUES-LACAN-XXIII.pdf
Lacan, J. (1976–1977). *Seminar XXIV, L'Insu que Sait de L'Une-Bévue S'Aile à Mourre* (1976–1977). [Online]. https://ecole-lacanienne.net/bibliolacan/stenotypies-version-j-l-et-non-j-l/
Lacan, J. (1991). *The Seminar of Jacques Lacan. Book I: Freud's Papers on Technique. 1953–1954*. W.W. Norton &Company.
Lacan, J. (1993). *The Psychoses. The Seminar of Jacques Lacan Book III, 1955–1956*. Routledge.
Lacan, J. (1997). *The Seminar of Jacques Lacan. Book VII: The Ethics of Psychoanalysis. 1959–1960*. W.W. Norton & Company.
Lacan, J. (1998). *The Seminar of Jacques Lacan. Book XX: Encore. On Feminine Sexuality, The Limits of Knowledge. 1972–1973*. W.W. Norton &Company.
Lacan, J. (2002). *The Seminar of Jacques Lacan XIII: The Object of Psychoanalysis*. Karnac.
Lacan, J. (2004). *Seminar XI. The Four Fundamental Concepts of Psycho-analysis*. Routledge.
Lacan, J. (2006). *Écrits*. W.W. Norton &Company.
Lacan, J. (2007). *The Seminar of Jacques Lacan. Book XVII The Other Side of Psychoanalysis*. W.W. Norton and Company.
Lacan, J. (2014). *Anxiety. The Seminar of Jacques Lacan Book X* (J-A. Miller, Ed.). Polity Press.
Lacan, J. (2015). *Transference: The Seminar of Jacques Lacan, Book VIII*. Polity.
Lacan, J. (2017). *The Seminar of Jacques Lacan. Book V: Formations of the Unconscious. 1957–1958*. Polity.

Miller, J. A. (2007). *La angustia—Introducción al Seminario X de Jacques Lacan*. Gredos.

Miller, J. A. (2008). Extimity. *The Symptom,* Issue 9. [Online]. https://www.lacan.com/symptom/extimity.html

Miller, J. A. (2021). Docile au Trans. *Lacan Quotidien., 928*(April), 3–18.

Millot, C. (1990). *Horsexe: Essay on Transsexuality*. Autononmedia.

Mitchell, J. (1982). `Introduction 1'. In J. Mitchell & J. Rose (Eds.), *Feminine Sexuality—Jacques Lacan and the école freudienne*. Norton-Pantheon.

Morel, G. (2000). *Sexual ambiguities*. The Centre for Freudian Analysis and Research Library CFAR.

Preciado, P. B. (2020). *Je suis um Monstre qui vous parle. Rapport pour une academie de psychanalystes*. Bernard Grasset.

Rose, J. (1986). *Sexuality in the Field of Vision*. Verso.

Roudinesco, E. (1997). *Jacques Lacan*. Columbia University Press.

Safatle, V. (2006). *A Paixão do Negativo: Lacan e a Dialética*. Editora UNESP.

Salecl, R. (2004). *On Anxiety*. Routledge.

Schuster, A. (2016). *The Trouble with Pleasure. Deleuze and Psychoanalysis*. The MIT Press.

Soler, C. (2014). *Lacanian Affects: The Function of Affect in Lacan's Work*. Routledge.

Van Haute, P. (2002). *Against Adaptation. Lacan's "Subversion" of the Subject. A Close Reading*. Other Press.

Voruz, V., & Wolf, B. (2007). *The Late Lacan, An Introduction*. State University of New York Press.

# 7

# Vibrating the Full-Void

Departing from Freud and Lacan's theories of anxiety—which see anxiety as an 'affect' and as 'an encounter with the Real'—we will now explore such interruption or rupture of the Symbolic net and the Imaginary frame that characterises anxiety via the concept of a '*vibrational body*'. Here I discuss, extrapolate and construct bridges through the dilemma between the abyss-within and possible horizons-beyond the subject as accounts of the Real.

How could we start thinking—and writing—about affect, about the Real, and about anxiety if what we are trying to reach is precisely the 'limits of language'? To anchor our thinking and to challenge the conceptualisation of the body in the context of anxiety I will discuss the notions of a 'vibrating body', the 'Plane' and the 'full-void' in the art work of Lygia Clark, which we started thinking about in the first chapter of this book. It is possible to make a parallel between Clark's 'abandonment of art' and such limits of language that are alive in the experience of anxiety as we will see in what follows. Clark's 'vibrational body', as observed by the Brazilian psychoanalyst Suely Rolnik (1989, 2000), not only pushes the definition of the status of the 'body' and affect in psychoanalysis as it offers a scope for an ontological debate over the status of the subject in and out of language. What Clark allows me to do is to travel beyond what


A. C. Minozzo, *Anxiety as Vibration*, Studies in the Psychosocial,
https://doi.org/10.1007/978-3-031-62856-6_7

she calls the 'Plane' of the Other, putting not only Oedipal sexual difference in check but also the barriers between psychoanalysis and an ethics of multiplicity instead of Lacan's ethics centred on the dialects of Desire—a move into the many beyond the two of the One, since this world is not one either, but many worlds at the same time.

In the next pages, Clark's work opens a discussion about affect, the Real, Oedipus and the limits of language; themes approached via an engagement with the interrogation: "*What can a body do?*" This puzzling question posited by Spinoza in the seventeenth century and picked up by Deleuze and Guattari from late 1960s is, we could easily agree, one that also moors the psychoanalytic clinic. From 'conversion hysteria' in Freud's couch to contemporary psychosomatic disease and at times 'unexplained' chronic illness, the body's capacity to produce symptoms, to react and to 'speak' appears as an important riddle of any analytical trajectory—and, as seen, in anxiety. The excessive, chaotic, unbound Real that is, across much of Freud and Lacan's work in need of 'castration', here will find ways into the *sinthôme* through a collectivising assemblage. Clark's vibrations 'beyond the Plane' allude to the realm of creativity and collectivity of affect that neither Freud nor Lacan articulate in their work of anxiety—but only hinted at in their 'vibrational moments'.

Following Guattari (2000), I agree that psychoanalysis needs an ethico-aesthetic reinvention; one that will move away from 'cultivating it' and its theories like an 'ornamental garden':

> In short, *the mythic and phantasmatic lure of psychoanalysis must be resisted, it must be played with, rather than cultivated and tended like an ornamental garden!* [my emphasis] Unfortunately, the psychoanalysts of today, more so than their predecessors, take refuge behind what one might call a 'structuralization' of unconscious complexes, which leads to dry theorisation and to insufferable dogmatism; also, their practice ends up impoverishing their treatments and produces a stereotyping which renders them insensible to the singular otherness [*alterité*] of their patients. (Guattari, 2000, p. 39)

Guattari is referring to Lacanians and the structuralist foundations of Lacan's theories of the unconscious that dominated his teaching specially during the 1960s. The trouble with this kind of psychoanalysis is, to Guattari, that it tries to encompass everything—all possibilities, all symptoms, all discourses—within its structural mapping (where the Other is the locus of all signifiers), making little space for the rise of and relationships among singular others. As such, working with this idea of vibration takes us to the realm of 'chaos', a threshold of creativity and immanence that posits an ontological and epistemological challenge to contemporary clinical practices. My intention is to discuss the limits and problems of a conceptualisation of the body and the Real through the dichotomy inherent in the Freudian and Lacanian 'drive'—a founding psychoanalytic concept that presupposes a division between language and flesh; between the realms of a castrating Symbolic and a chaotic body. Agreeing with Braidotti (2006), I see one central problem with the psychoanalytic theory of the drive in Lacan as that it relies on a Hegel-inherited negativity of desire and a dialectics of 'sexual difference', structuring subjectivity into a nuclear and out-dated family drama.

In what follows, we will dive deeper into the world of chaos by taking not just Guattari and Deleuze as companions, but also Spinoza, whose *Ethics* can illuminate the vibrating possibilities of anxiety. Art practice, here, will be crucial to our push beyond critique and towards creativity in the field of psy-care, unfolding mainstream theories through vibration.

## A Horizon-beyond the Plane of Oedipus

One of the central critiques to the project of psychoanalysis conferred by Gilles Deleuze and Félix Guattari in their seminal *Capitalism and Schizophrenia* two-volume work, from 1972 and 1980 respectively, concerns the reactionary politics of the psychoanalytic clinic, from its institutional arrangements to the politics of its assumed subject. Perhaps, we could argue, whilst not a direct feminist intervention on the psychoanalytic model and its ties with a patriarchal arrangement of power in social bond and psychic life, *Anti-Oedipus*, does, however, manage to challenge very clearly one problem relevant to what we are looking into: the question of 'excess' in light of 'castration'. Excess, in this case, both as what exceeds meaning and as what accumulates in the form of a 'libidinal energy' and the mechanism of its destinies according to Freud, post-Freudians and Lacan. What is described as a 'molar' and 'neurotic' tree-like unconscious is contrasted, famously, with a 'molecular', 'rhizomatic' (Deleuze & Guattari, 1983, 1987) and thus multiple version not bound to a Symbolic cut guaranteed by what Lacan calls the 'Father function' of Oedipus' castrating moral necessity.

The Freudian Oedipal resolution was absorbed into Lacanian structuralism.[1] So, instead of its dissolution resulting in the Super-Ego, Ego and Id, we will then speak of language and the effects of the signifier on the mythical pre-Symbolic subject (the one represented by the delta in the bottom right of the Lacanian Graph of Desire). The entrance into the Symbolic, thus, has a structuring effect akin to an invitation into neurosis. Upon failure to joining 'civilisation and its discontents' we find psychosis.[2] Yet, a philosophical enquiring of the psychoanalytic subject here leads me to the following question: is there anything beyond psychosis outside this patriarchal conception of the possibilities for the subject? What are the grounds for rupture in the clinic? Is everything that aligns to a Real outside of the scope of the Other necessarily on the side of psychosis? The close readings of Freud and Lacan suggest that anxiety remains at an impasse in the clinic: it points to a rupture, but the rupture was repeatedly circumscribed within an Oedipal alienating frame, although not always limited to it (the vibrational moments in Freud and Lacan's theories of anxiety attesting as much). Lygia Clark's push beyond the Plane, as I will argue in what follows, inspires an ethics of multiplicity that works itself against the dominance of the Oedipal model of the unconscious.

What I propose in what follows is that there is plenty there beyond psychosis, escaping language, escaping Oedipal binaries and escaping castration—and through the experience of the affect of anxiety we are in touch with this excess that is both radical and expanding as well as

[1] In Seminar III, Lacan teaches clearly that "every analytic phenomenon, every phenomenon that comes from the analytic field, from the analytic discovery from what we are dealing with in symptoms and neurosis, is structured like a language" (Lacan, 1993, p. 167), as such the Other as the locus of all signifiers is anchored through the Law-of-the-Father that gives consistency, according to this version of Lacan, to the unconscious.

[2] However, in regard to this point—the primacy of this entrance into the Symbolic to the formation of the Lacanian subject, the unconscious and its relevant structure—we must never forget the clear non-pathologising, therefore radical on its own terms, take on these outcomes, or the non-hierarchical relation between neurosis and psychosis in the Lacanian psychoanalytic tradition.

paralysing and excruciating. This 'surplus' in anxiety marks the rhythm of what Deleuze and Guattari named as 'becomings' (*devenir*). Anxiety is what persists, insists and opens up to a possibility in subjective experience directly emerged from the vibrational body facing the limits of language. To arrive at this understanding we must, however, salvage this 'vibrating body' from the enthralment of the Other, Oedipus and the Symbolic, thus, of patriarchy and its ideological allies. Such endeavour consists in rescuing Spinoza's affective 'surplus'—noticeably an important influence on Deleuzian and Guattarian thought—in Freud's very early and very late writings on anxiety, and Lacan's later teachings and what they may mean to a theory of anxiety. This reading also throws some light on Lacan's very complicated late teachings and assigns, therefore, a political potency to the ubiquitous and necessary experience of anxiety. An experience central not only to the very development of psychoanalysis as well as to twentieth century psychiatric diagnosis and the psycho-political arrangement of contemporary late-capitalism.

The Oedipal foundations of sexual difference is a matter that has historically permeated the debates between an 'essentialist' current in feminist thought, specially of 1970s second wave feminism and the queer interventions of the 1990s. Antoinette Fouque, a member of the French *Mouvement de libération des femmes* (MLF), for example, a follower of Lacan and Irigaray and companion of Serge Leclaire and Monique Wittig, proposes as part of the group *Psychanalyse et Politique* a return to sexual difference from the perspective of women. Fouque (1995), as found in the collection *Il y a deux sexes: essais de féminologie. 1989–1995*, believed in the 'feminine libido', which was not reliant on the phallic dominance of Freudian and Lacanian theory, which she understood to only account for the sex of the 'one'—men. This feminine libido was incarnated in the experience of symbolic gestation, which she saw as offering an ethical position of subjective production, alliance and alterity against the patriarchal 'brotherhood' of post-1968 France.[3] This symbolic function of the mother was her way into a psychoanalysis of the 'two' sexes, rather than the 'one' of its Oedipal matrix. Fouque, as well as Irigaray, was an

[3] Symbolic gestation being echoed also in Bracha Ettinger's (2019) more recent work, addressing the concept of *co-poiesis*.

important figure of inspiration for the development of a branch of Italian feminism that is concerned with sexual difference—with thinkers such as Luisa Muraro, Lia Cigarini and Lea Melandri.[4]

In Italy, however, the feminist movements, which were, in the 1970s, close to Marxist and psychoanalytic ideas, take 'difference' away from only the difference between two sexes (male and female), anchoring it as a difference within oneself (Zamboni, 2019). Difference, in this tradition of feminist psychoanalytic thought, is what guarantees a critique of the depoliticising absorption into the status quo, therefore into patriarchy, as a 'piece' of its puzzle without real emancipation.[5] A plural, multiple version of sexual difference, which takes it away from the Oedipal inscription and its consequential dialectic framing upon a 'phallogocentric' referential, and into the realm of a 'nomadic subjectivity' is Braidotti's contribution to the field, since the early 1990s. She holds on to sexual difference as a significant tool for political analysis, revisiting the topic in light of contemporary political, ecological, scientific and social debates, whilst maintaining a dialogue with contemporary feminists that do not consider sexual difference as a conceptual problem for feminism at all (such as 'post-Deleuzian' feminists Moira Gatens & Genevieve Lloyd, 1999; or Claire Colebrook, 2000). Whilst this book is not focused on resolving the vast discussion of sexual difference within feminist theory, nor on offering a detailed genealogy of this debate, it is important to mention how the reduction of difference into a binary is still characteristic of contemporary Lacanian works. Without dismissing the reality of patriarchy, oppression and exploitation in concrete but also in its psychological and unconscious traumatic consequences, an understanding of difference that moves beyond the Plane of Oedipus also allows us to think of the Real and its irruptions in anxiety as unbound by the One of the Other and pertaining to the sphere of affect that is creative, collective and in movement (rather than a rupture limited to the side of psychosis).

Alenka Zupančič (2017), an important contemporary feminist scholar, defends sexual difference as an equation of logics: we can only have

[4] Lia Cigarini's 1995 *La Politica del Desiderio* promotes more clearly an affirmative and productive political landscape for feminist constructions departing from the point of difference.

[5] A view that resonates a way of thinking of feminism in alliance with Critical Theory.

difference and the failure of encounter, the gap in subjectivity, if we set out a system of two. Zupančič is not, however, being simplistic, essentialist or anti-feminist with this remark about her defence of sexual difference as a concept; quite the opposite, her argument is that only within such a logic of two (which does not have to do with gender, or 'real' 'man' or 'woman', but with subjective positions), can we account for a power relation of inequality and oppression. This is, without a doubt, a powerful and important point. The 'One' has oppressed the 'Not-one', this 'Not-all' that does not (think to) have the phallus; and the Imaginary-Symbolic repertoire of modern humanism foreclosed the Real and any experience as part of a 'common' (Federici, 2019, 2020). The calculation of unequal status, for Zupančič (2017), needs this artifice of difference. Following Copjec, she argues that 'sexual difference', in Lacan, is a logic of two that allows us to see the power relation and the inconsistency that crosses the subject (a difference not between 'man' and 'woman', but a difference within 'oneself'). It is her understanding that gender theory took this difference to the level of the surface, rather than depth, calling for a multiplicity that does not account for such 'difference', or the 'gap' that produces the relation between the two.[6] Her argument, as she explains:

> goes—both methodologically and ideologically—against the grain of the "times we live in," refusing to abandon the construction site in favour of more polished "conceptual products," "services," or "singular experiences." [The pages that follow] grew out of a double conviction: first, that in psychoanalysis sex is above all a *concept* that formulates a persisting contradiction of reality. And, second, that this contradiction cannot be circumscribed or reduced to a secondary level (as a contradiction between already well-established entities/beings), but is—*as a contradiction*—involved in the very structuring of these entities, in their very being. In this precise sense, sex is of ontological relevance: not as an ultimate reality, but as an inherent twist, or stumbling block, of reality. (Zupančič, 2017, p. 3)

[6] Another important feminist critique of the Deleuze-Guattari machinic model that takes sexual difference away from centre stage is Luce Irigaray's, whose "critique of Deleuze is radical: she points out that the dispersal of sexuality into a generalized 'becoming' results in undermining the feminist claims to a redefinition of the female subject" (Braidotti, 2011, p. 38).

'Sex', according to this argument, guarantees this 'too-muchness' of the abyss-within, an understanding that needs to be salvaged from the full trust in the signifier that tries to encapsulate identity in new names and definitions for such inconsistency. This view, whilst radical in its own manner, seems to be still thinking of psychoanalysis as 'an ornamental garden' (Guattari, 2000) that needs to be well kept rather than transformed with time. This view—sexual difference or barbarism/neoliberalism (or worse, in Millot and Morel: sexual difference or psychosis/madness)—can easily turn ideological and sour.

Such a view echoes Žižek's (2004) criticism of post-Deleuzian work, which he holds as not accounting for any antagonism inherent to subjectivity, and fitting in very nicely with neoliberal accumulation and eternity of production.[7] He slips, however, when asserting that the proliferation of gender and sexual identities in the twenty-first century (including within it all expressions of affirmation of non-conforming identities, such as trans) are all ideological escapes of such antagonism. Žižek writes, in a very polemical essay for *The Philosophical Salon*, in 2016, that "difference 'in itself' is thus not symbolic-differential, but real-impossible—something that eludes and resists the symbolic grasp" (Žižek, 2016).[8] Whilst this affirmation is fine and 'sound' in terms of its faithfulness to Lacanian

---

[7] When Braidotti articulates this ethical possibility in *Transpositions*, she mobilises the concepts of *bios* and *zoe*, as elaborated by Agamben and further extended into her post-humanist feminist model of immanence. This is a theoretical artifice that is invaluable for the non-liberalism of the concept of multiplicity—a pitfall of some post-Deleuzian works that see an infinite proliferation of positivity within one's reach, seeing 'desire' as production and infinite but thwarting Deleuze and Guattari's unequivocal anti-capitalist and ecological argument into simplistic ideas such as 'accelerationism' (Williams & Srnicek, 2013). In *zoe*, Braidotti acknowledges the historical and political mechanisms of isolation, destruction and alienation of this 'type' of life—dividing Life into 'life' and 'bare life', as per Agamben's elaboration in *Homo Sacer* (1995). Yet, "Bradotti brings *zoe* in from the cold, foregrounding this brutal inhuman force as a productive category" (Baraitser, 2010, p. 127) instead, seeing it as the key out of a subjective arrangement and biopolitical organisation reliant on a binary constitution of 'sameness'. The ecofeminist ethics proposed by Braidotti in this work are anchored thus "in terms of *zoe*, or generative, non-logocentric life: a micro-politics of affective becomings" (Braidotti, 2006, p. 131). In other words, by unfastening a "joint reliance on the phallic signifier, i.e. the political economy of Sameness and of its specular, binary and constitutive 'Others'" (Braidotti, 2006, p. 130), it is possible to take an ethical position "as a non-unitary, nomadic feminist and accountable subject [which] facilitates this bond of both empathy and responsibility towards non-human others" (Braidotti, 2006, p. 130).

[8] Sabsay (2016), for instance, discusses at length the problems of the question of difference and the liberalisation of sexual identities globally in more grounded and responsible ways than Žižek.

concepts, it seems to be a view that 'tends to the ornamental garden' of psychoanalysis, pruning its concepts for theoretical fruits that look more perfect—a move that sounds, to me at least, exactly like the blind-faith in the signifier that this rather conservative approach tries to antagonise. The 'phallus', in this approach, is maintained as essential, making of 'feminine' and 'masculine' sexuation a conceptual binary that follows unquestioned. The fact that a 'binary' is the only guarantor of any ethical probity (with 'lack' in its centre) is not only problematic on the surface (implying that calling masculine and feminine something else, something 'neutral', A or B, would resolve it); rather, it is more complicated in depth.[9] This binary that sustains lack is problematic in its very principle, following the dynamics of 'difference and separation' that Denise Ferreira da Silva (2016) connects so astutely with the onto-epistemological pillars of colonialism, patriarchy and human exceptionalism. In defence of a collective entanglement, she writes:

> Without separability, knowing and thinking can no longer be reduced to determinacy in the Cartesian distinction of mind/body (in which the latter has the power of determination) or the Kantian formal reduction of knowing to a kind of efficient causality. Without separability, sequentiality (Hegel's ontoepistemological pillar) can no longer account for the many

[9] Lorenzo Chiesa (2016) wrote a whole book exploring this question of the 'two' in Lacan. In *The Not-Two Logic and God in Lacan*, Chiesa argues that through his study of Seminar XX, which he sees as one of "the Seminars revolving around the axiom 'There is no sexual relationship', and perhaps the most inconclusive, it also undoubtedly remains to date the most commented-on and liable to misinterpretations (due often to a lack of involvement with earlier works). In short, such mistaken appraisals tend to share an identification of woman, who for Lacan emerges as a singular, nonuniversalizable une femme, with The Other. This view is especially confusing when voiced from allegedly feminist quarters: Woman as The Other supposedly irreducible to castration—namely, in the end, as the unity of substance of the classical metaphysical God—corresponds in fact for Lacan to nothing other than the illusory counterpart of the evanescent object through which man enjoys woman in his fundamental fantasy. We therefore need to interrupt this short circuit. The unbinding of a woman from The Other will also provide us with the right coordinates of feminine non-phallic jouissance, a supplementary enjoyment that is, however, linked to structure as its not-all, and thus does not prevent the Other sex from enjoying phallically" (Chiesa, 2016, p. xx). Chiesa moves further away from Žižek/ Zupančič's reliance on sexual difference by exploring further the 'non-phallic jouissance' of the Other/feminine, however, assigning this jouissance to the realm of asexuality—again, a troublesome point from a feminist perspective. 'Non-phallic' jouissance is inscribed within a dialectical relation with phallic jouissance, in other words, bound to a relation with this universal. Whilst this is 'correct' as an archaeology of terms within Lacanian archives, it fails to engage with contemporary life and ethical demands.

> ways in which humans exist in the world, because self-determination has a very limited region (spacetime) for its operation. When nonlocality guides our imaging of the universe, difference is not a manifestation of an unresolvable estrangement, but the expression of an elementary entanglement. (Ferreira da Silva, 2016, p. 65)

Fittingly, when contemporary philosophers and psychoanalysts call for a move beyond the colonial unconscious—as Braidotti, but also Preciado (2020) and Rolnik (2015, 2019) do—multiplicity, immanence and becoming-with are the grounds for conceiving an idea of subjectivity and the unconscious based on an ecosophy (Guattari, 2000). By ecosophy, following Guattari's method in *The Three Ecologies* (2000), I mean a social, ecological and psychic entanglement of the subject, and an onto-ethical framework that departs from such entanglement, rather than the post-Kantian distance from the world. Going back to Lygia Clark, the phantasmatics of the body, the 'full-void' and their vibrations in collective *poieses* are elaborations that speak closely to 'difference' without 'separability' and, rather, differences within multiplicities.

Moving beyond the binary of sexual difference—taking seriously the mechanisms of production and reproduction that engender this still limited Oedipal and phallic arrangement, namely a universalist modern humanism anchored in dominance and extraction—is a task that resonates with Deleuze and Guattari's work since *Anti-Oedipus*.[10] The critique of such unitarian and universal points of referencing that are assumed as structuring is at the core of Guattari's clinical, theoretical and political project, since "Guattari contests the unitary, homogeneous and authoritarian model of organisation, and privileges instead a type of system with multiple, a-centred connections" (Sauvagnargues, 2016, p. 141). The mechanism and the machine are the conceptual resources mobilised by Deleuze and Guattari to trace the possibilities of becoming, taking, as it is well known, psychoanalysis for a radical and yet conservative praxis, rescuing it from Oedipus (or the structure of production and reproduction of the One in the colonial and patriarchal capitalist delirium).

---

[10] Or the bi-univocity, or the turning bivocal of what is polyvocal, as per Guattari (2006), as the movement that dividualises or estranges our experience of anxiety.

In *The Machinic Unconscious*, from 1979, Guattari "proposes a 'machinic' unconscious and not a structural one, an unconscious populated to be sure with images and words, but also with the mechanisms of reproductions of these images and words (Guattari, 1995b). This unconscious is thus not representative or expressive, but productive" (Sauvagnargues, 2016, p. 153). There is something here I hold on to in terms of the ethical and feminist potency of Freudian and Lacanian psychoanalysis, which, in a certain way, is characterised by a movement of attempting to trace the mechanisms of becoming, situated, however, in its own contextual blindness. Juliet Mitchel, in her introduction to the volume on *Feminine Sexuality* co-authored with Jaqueline Rose in 1982, writes very succinctly and with clarity about the somewhat 'post-humanist' potency in psychoanalysis, for it pulls back the curtain of the mirage of the subject:

> The humanistic conception of mankind assumes that the subject exists from the beginning. At least by implication ego psychologists, object-relations theorists and Kleinians base themselves on the same premise. For this reason, Lacan considers that in the last analysis, they are more ideologues than theorists of psychoanalysis. In the Freud that Lacan uses, neither the unconscious nor sexuality can in any degree be pre-given facts, they are constructions, that is, they are objects with histories and the human subject itself is only formed within these histories…This immediately establishes the framework within which the whole question of female sexuality can be understood. As Freud puts it: `In conformity with its peculiar nature, psychoanalysis does not try to describe what a woman is—that would be a task it could scarcely perform—but sets about enquiring *how she comes into being*.' (Mitchell, 1982, p. 4)

In this sense, Freudian and Lacanian psychoanalysis set out to elucidate the mechanisms of the machine that is the unconscious, with limits, of course, but still stirring a revolution within hegemonic onto-epistemic ideals of their time. The subject, therefore, is not 'pre-given', but a coming into being, or, rather, a 'coming into becoming'. Freud and Lacan, at the very least, lift the veil of the alienation that is neurosis or the entrance into the Symbolic and succumbing to the Law. Preciado, in closing remarks of his published speech addressed to the École de la cause

Freudienne de Paris from November 2019, calls for a revolutionary mutation of psychoanalysis, one that addresses and moves beyond its patriarchal and colonial presuppositions.[11] For Preciado, the answers to our situated and contemporary ecological, social, political as well as epistemological, scientific and ontological matters are not to be found in reading and re-reading Freud and Lacan (or tending to the ornamental garden), rather, being faithful to the revolution in thought inaugurated by Freud means to 'decolonise the unconscious' (Preciado, 2020).[12]

As Braidotti (2006) acknowledges in *Transpositions*, but also as any attentive reader of Deleuze and Guattari can grasp, Spinoza's monism and theory of affects, that inspired them greatly, allows a logic in which 'sexual difference' does not need to be anchoring of subjectivity as such. We don't need to think through Oedipal sexual difference and the mirage of a One that is All (following the Freudian myth in *Totem and Taboo*), nor of the Not-All as its binary opposition, always caught in the Master's eyes; rather, it is a matter of understanding all subjective arrangements as necessarily not-all, since 'all' does not exist except in an ideological onto-epistemic mirage.[13] This view contradicts that of Alenka Zupančič (2017, 2019), for example, as mentioned previously, that a system of two, regulated by the Phallic Law, is necessary in order to account for dominance, and therefore for patriarchal violence to be broader, an argument carved out of mathematical logics, which nonetheless turns a blind eye to its own violent reproductions.

---

[11] He writes: "*Nous avons besoin d'une transition de la clinique. Cela ne peut se faire que par une mutation révolutionnaire de la psychanalyse et un dépassement critique de ses présupposés patriarcat-coloniaux*" (Preciado, 2020, pp. 54–55).

[12] Elisabeth Roudinesco, the grand historian of French psychoanalysis and biographer of Lacan, called the book 'unconvincing' in her review for the French newspaper *Le Monde*. One aspect Roudinesco did not enjoy in particular was how the author, Preciado, drew too much on his personal experience of transition. The title and subtitle of her article read: "*Le philosophe trans s'appuie sur son expérience pour appeler à « décoloniser » l'inconscient. Sans convaincre*". In English, "the trans philosopher bases himself on his own experience to call for a 'decolonisation' of the unconscious. Without convincing" (Roudinesco, 2020).

[13] Being very precise, we could accept that the 'phallus', as it is delineated in Lacanian teachings, appears as this mythical and at the same time empty signified that demarcates the territory of such an onto-epistemic mirage.

## The Vibrational Body and Anxiety, an Encounter Beyond the Plane

Whilst Deleuze and Guattari were sharp critics of psychoanalysis, Guattari's later works curiously turned to Freud's early works and the notion of libido beyond the constraints of an Oedipalised subject—which are systematised in this early theory of anxiety. In June 1983, Guattari was part of a colloquium in Cerisy, France, about the work of the physical chemist Ilya Prigogine where he presented a paper entitled 'Semiotic Energetics'. This paper later composed his book *Schizoanalytic Cartographies*, from 1989, and marks what Watson (2009) points at being his 'return to Freud' via a rather cryptic formulation of energetics (Guattari, 1989). Central to his argument is the understanding that Freud's early texts gave more emphasis to the 'energetic' factor of an essential 'libidinal energy' that was side-lined in his second topography. In this sense, what Freud's project envisaged, writes Guattari, was "to establish passageways between sexual libido and effects of meaning [...] [in] his initial hypothesis of an energy whose effects were simultaneously physical and psychic" (Guattari & Rolnik, 2007, p. 394). However, such energy metaphors (which Guattari found in the pre-psychoanalytic texts and letters to Fliess) were lost in the second model of the psyche, resulting in what Guattari diagnosed as "the psychoanalytic movement never stop[ping] submitting the concept of libidinal energy to a wide variety of treatments in order to try to dominate the theoretical scandal of which it is the vehicle" (Guattari & Rolnik, 2007, p. 394). Freud, post-Freudians and also Lacanian structuralism thus committed to "nothing more nor less than its [libidinal energy's] virtually total liquidation in the form of a chain of signifiers" (Guattari & Rolnik, 2007, p. 394). The Symbolic order, charged with social, subjective and epistemological constructions of the colonial patriarchal arrangement, gives consistency to a clinic that is founded upon a surplus—the unconscious—yet articulated through the very motor that subsumes the rupture, or the potency of the flux of becomings of this very excess.

The principles of their schizoanalysis and a conceptualisation of desire as production broke away from the psychoanalytic focus on the 'individual', favouring a "collective economy, collective assemblages of desire and of subjectivity that can be individualised in some circumstances or some social contexts" (Guattari & Rolnik, 2007, p. 343). This intrinsically political view of desire, the unconscious and subjectivity, therefore was fruitful to feminist thinkers. Feminist scholars have dug into the work of Deleuze and Guattari and their schizoanalytic model to challenge the psychoanalytic understanding that language, or the Symbolic, was structuring. Bracha Ettinger, for instance, presents an affirmative, or generative, matrix for subjective variation in her 'metramorphosis' (Ettinger, 2006) alive in her painting and clinic. Elizabeth Grosz and Rosi Braidotti, on the other hand, flesh out the philosophical underpinnings to an affirmative understanding of desire in debates on the ontological, ethical and political concepts that permeate subjectivity, materiality, 'scientific' biological discourses and technology (Grosz, 2008, 2017; Braidotti, 2017). What I propose here, as a small gesture into this debate, however, is to go back to Spinoza, the Dutch seventeenth century philosopher who influenced Deleuze and, later Guattari, greatly in their understanding of the body and affect. What I intend is to map the possibilities that Spinoza's monism offers to Lygia Clark's full-void, phantasmatic, 'vibrating body'. More specifically, we will be looking for a possible transindividual connection in his *Ethics*, and a political or collective linkage of the understanding of affects, symptoms and subjective formation that is present in Spinoza's ontology as a ground to think, with Lygia Clark, of what is the horizon-beyond the Plane.

A zigzag of subject, affect and conditions of subjectivity framed by ideology in the social bond is present my psychosocial or critical reading of psychoanalysis. According to such approach, a 'subjective truth' occurs both in the dynamic of symptom formation and the singular function of symptoms. This is Lacan's clear contribution to clinical work: situating the subject and symptoms, by identifying their function within a particular cartography he called the Symbolic. Yet, beyond a structural focus on meaning and deciphering of the symptom, Freud's very early 'energetic' grounds for a bodily source of anxiety see anxiety as an affect of surplus: it emerges when something in the material experience of the body or in the realm of 'ideas' limits the flux of the libidinal energy that characterises the life of the body (in a Bergsonian sense of a 'life' being a tendency that "'unfolds' that which is folded in matter" (Grosz, 2007, p. 295)).

Spinoza's conception of nature, human existence and the mind are detailed in his *Ethics*, where a view of an infinite substance (which he calls God) that is constantly modified and has different attributes opens a way for the debate on possibility and flux of said substance and the differences in such attributes. In Part I, Proposition V, Spinoza states that "there cannot exist in the universe two or more substances having the same nature or attribute". In this sense, nature is understood for its differential values, not of different substances as such (as put in a Note to Proposition X, Part I "there is but one substance in the universe, and that it is absolutely infinite") but of its different modes. Whilst God is an infinity of possibility, a body is a 'finite mode' of expression of this substance, Part II, Def. I. (Curley, 1994). This focus on 'differential values' and, thus, a disequilibrium as a structural necessity is what allows Spinoza to shed light on this complicated relation between 'mind' and 'body' (Kordela, 2007). His monism did not simply clear the slate of any difference; rather, it speaks of 'thoughts' and 'bodies' as different in attributes and nature, thus, in 'value'. A surplus in this differential arrangement is evident in the following passage from Part I, Definition II "A thing is called 'finite after its kind'\ when it can be limited by another thing of the same nature; for instance, a body is called finite because we always conceive another greater body. So, also, a thought is limited by another thought, but a body is not limited by thought, nor a thought by body". In this sense something of the existence of the body cannot be grasped by thoughts in the same way that thoughts do not find total representation in the body. This very simple conceptual interpretation of a 'surplus' when it comes to the subject as a 'being' of concomitant dissonant values speaks to the Freudian earlier conception of anxiety as an excess that finds no grounds in either the 'body' or the 'mind'.

This conception of surplus here also brings another layer of complication to that notion of 'excess' immanent to language, or to the Symbolic in Lacan's early works. Lacanian scholars, and noticeably Žižek (1992), stress how psychoanalysis should not take the patient's complaint at face value, following Freud, a fair and radical point, especially in regards to therapeutic practices that reject the unconscious and serve well the hegemonic ideology of the contemporary late-capitalism. Instead, psychoanalysis would then look for the 'excess' of meaning in what the patient comes to say, or the "surplus of what is effectively said, not the intended message, but the message in its true, inverted form" (Kordela, 2007, p. 7). This version of the Real, in Lacan's terms, aside from being contested by contemporary literature on his later teachings (Miller, 2003; Soler, 2014; Schuster, 2016), still ascribes psychoanalysis to a mode of interpretation of symptoms that can be radical as a "new mode of semiotization of subjectivity" inaugurated by Freud's work with patients diagnosed as hysterics, but still needs further breaks "with the universes of reference" (Guattari & Rolnik, 2007) it reproduces. Going beyond 'interpretation' (as Clark did in *Structuring of the Self*) means, for Guattari, going beyond the 'power' of an analyst and also of 'words' within their universal referential (Other), meant to embark on 'analytic revolutions' that break away with predetermined or pre-inscribed "stratified modes of subjectivation" not solely bound to the clinical encounter. He writes of this radical commitment with the surplus as being part of "modes of asignifying rupture, which appeared simultaneously in literature, Surrealism, painting, and so on" (Guattari & Rolnik, 2007, p. 381). Instead of a 'rest' to what we can 'think' of, this excess in anxiety could be thought of in relation to what Guattari calls 'chaos'. Chaos speaks closely to the full-void, addressing precisely a horizon-beyond the abyss-within.

To Guattari, 'a body' is a reality that presents itself in constant tension between the 'chaotic' accumulation and flux of libidinal energy and what harnesses it, either allowing new conjunctions to emerge or posing a limit (Berardi, 2015). The contour of a body marked by words, words of a Symbolic realm structured within a colonial patriarchal modus operandi, would suggest a circularity of the repetitions under the logic of the Death Drive (Khanna, 2003). For such libidinal flow evident in Freud's very early texts, so cherished by Guattari, to carry an affirmative character, what needs to be redefined is precisely the mythical pre-subjective state that Lacan (and not Freud) granted to be a 'negativity' (at least in early and mid-life works). It is Hegel's influence in the accounting of time and history that fostered the privileging of a Symbolic that could not change effectively, and so limited the very notions of creativity, singularity, potency and affirmation (Braidotti, 2017). Contrary to superficial readings, the Spinozist twist of Deleuze and Guattari's project was not offering a view of the subject as having a 'reservoir of positivity' to start with that is then 'lost' as we encounter the mad-bad-sad Oedipal Capitalist order. In Guattari's elaboration on the notion of 'chaos' in *Chaosmosis*, 1992, and in the collection *Chaosophy*, 1995, we see this 'libidinal energy' that Freud observes to be floating through the body in the earlier texts on anxiety not as an 'originative beginning', but as a middle, a flux that breaks with the duality body/word and focuses on the 'threshold', the 'frontier' (Guattari, 2009). As such, this frontier, the a-signifying ruptures of the unconscious, should not be interpreted out of such reservoir, rather, they should be mobilised into *poiesis*.[14] A tension, a threshold, a zone of inventiveness, transformation and creativity are, in this sense, of the level of 'chaos'.

Spinozist lenses here reveal then that the 'affirmation' is a matter of difference, of the surplus generated in the 'middle', as life goes on rather than a power that was there and is then 'lost' by our entrance into culture. In this sense, thinking of anxiety as the affect of affirmation (thus, difference and transformation rather than repetition and resistance) also speaks to the trope of finding in melancholia and therefore in 'failed mourning' an identification with what is lost as a way to resist power. Butler's (1997) work in *The Psychic Life of Power* (which draws the line between Hegel,

[14] Poiesis has an interesting route in the thinking of Guattari all the way into contemporary feminist Post-human thinking that is worth mentioning. Guattari presents in *The Three Ecologies* and also in *Chaosmosis*—the 1992 compilation where Guattari is influenced by the biological theory of Francisco Varela—the notion of 'autopoiesis'. Varela and Maturana, Chilean philosophers, proposed in the early 1970s that cells and the life that extends from this minimal 'machine' operate through a process of continuous self-production, or an autopoiesis. Cells are not a given, rather, they are production. In his clinical work at La Borde, Guattari sees a continuous production of subjectivity unfolding, writing that "we are not confronted with a subjectivity given as in-itself, but with processes of the realization of autonomy, or of autopoiesis (in a somewhat different sense from the one Francisco Varela gives this term)" (Guattari, 1995a, p. 7). However, he pushed Varela's ideas further, subverting them in an important manner by calling for a 'collective' autopoiesis, or for a subjective production "beyond Varela's characterization of machinic autopoiesis as unitary individuation, with neither input or output" (Guattari, 1995a, p. 42), proposing rather "a more collective machinism without delimited unity, whose autonomy accommodates diverse mediums of alterity" (Guattari, 1995a, p. 42). Rosi Braidotti (2006) is also attuned to this detail, interpreting that Guattari paid attention to "the non-human parts of human subjectivity, which is not an anti-humanist position but merely the acknowledgement that subjectivity does not and need not coincide with either the notion of the individual or that of person" (Braidotti, 2006, p. 125). The production, actualization and invention in this process concern the subject beyond itself, in a constant, meaning that "autopoiesis is processual creativity" (Braidotti, 2006, p. 126). More recently, Donna Haraway (2016) thinks of poiesis under the prism of the Gaia hypothesis as proposed by Lynn Margulis, adding the nuance of 'sympoiesis' over the term 'autopoiesis' to stress the becoming-with characteristic of life in its collectivity rather than individuality. Poiesis (co/auto/symp) is at the heart of Clark's 'vibrational' technique.

Nietzsche, Freud and Foucault) presupposed some linearity of time even if in an 'ideal' form. Also radical in its critique of identitarian oppression, the focus on 'loss'—either of what was there and then was lost or even pushing it into the loss of what 'could be there' but was not allowed to—does not break with the transcendental universal of the Other and time in its struggle for recognition. In this sense, it will also not break away from the pre-eminence of language as located in the Other, or the patriarchal-colonial Symbolic and the consequent dialectics of recognition therein inscribed.[15] To put it differently, following the vocabulary of my engagement with Lygia Clark, we will still be harnessing multiplicity and the full-void into the realm of the One of Sameness. An exploration of what lies beyond the logic of patriarchy, thus, an 'excess' that is produced by the difference of the 'middle' that is alive in the affect of anxiety proves to be more fruitful to thought.

To connect this differential production of the 'middle' with the libido of early-Freud's 'energetic' flows, another core concept from Spinoza's *Ethics* is helpful: conatus. From the Latin for a tendency to 'strive', Spinoza defines it as "Each thing, as far as it can by its own power, strives to persevere in its being", Proposition VI, Part III (Curley, 1994). Not simply carrying on 'being', or self-preservation, but also having their 'power of action increased', is what Spinoza defines for the conative quality of bodies. This 'affirmative' tendency is necessarily 'shared' or 'collective', relational instead of self-referential, once it is related to the increase

---

[15] Butler's (1997) work, as well as the work of Jessica Benjamin (1998), Amy Allen (2015) and other contemporary feminist theorists who engage with Critical Theory, powerfully situates not only gender but political subjectivity in the cracks of a Hegelian negativity and dialectics. Psychic life here is modelled onto a frame that is in line with an Idealist transcendental, posing in the unconscious, sexuality, the drive and the Real (the psychoanalytic sites of 'rupture') a potency for movement and emancipation. In this sense, performativity and becoming align in their opening to something new, to transformation (Tuhkanen, 2009). However, if the clinic, as most of Lacan's early and mid-life works encompass, remains at the level of a dialectical enunciation and recognition via interpretation, rupture does not yet foster any affective novel modes of living and relating; rather, it alleviates suffering by alleviating its pressure onto the status quo. 'Spitting on Hegel', to me, entails a fundamentally decolonial effort to multiply universalising transcendentals into plural immanent matrices. Transformation, in this sense, still locks possibility on the eyes of the hegemonic discourse, rather than unfolding materiality beyond a system of 'two', and the consequential Oedipal inscription of the drive, desire and demand, as clinical reality often presents as a necessity. The 'transversal' clinic, as Guattari (2015) practiced at La Borde, aimed to mobilise chaos precisely into an 'assemblage' that is collective and situated.

or decrease of the capacity to be affected and to affect other bodies. His ontology thus proposes that we share the same substance which is in the world in different and differential modalities. In sharp contrast with the negativity of desire (not to mention its connection with a 'need' and 'demand' that subscribe it to the phallic function in Lacan's early teachings), what moves our lives is not a repetition of negativity, but an affirmative tendency to produce difference anchored in this 'surplus' that is an excess of the order of experience. In this sense, conatus is more akin to Freud's early texts that attribute value to such libidinal energy that is 'converted' into various symptoms or into anxiety.

For Berardi, the answer to this ethical riddle is in *co-poiesis*, creating together something new and of the order of sensibility. Here, echoing Lygia Clark's method in *Structuring of the Self* very beautifully. Poetry can attune subjectivity to the order of Chaos, or "an environment that is too complex to be decoded by our available explanatory frames, an environment in which fluxes circulate too quickly for our minds to elaborate" (Berardi, 2018, p. 39). Such a definition of chaos, for Berardi, makes explicit the rhythmic encounter with the 'vibration of the world', whilst "poetry is an attempt to tune into this cosmic vibration, this temporal vibration that is coming and coming" (Berardi, 2018, p. 17).

'Difference' and 'antagonism' are two philosophical notions of particular importance when mapping the Clark's full-void 'vibrational body' in relation to surplus. A vibrational body, thus, connotes a surplus beyond the limits of Symbolic language in its Oedipal foundation, a surplus at stake in the formulations of anxiety seen both in Freud and Lacan, but which I am trying to mobilise psycho-politically (also out of a Modern humanist and patriarchal matrix). Surplus, in a Spinozist understanding, presupposes difference (such as the full-void). So instead of thinking of an ontology of the subject in which affirmation is without 'antagonism' (as Žižek, 2010, would put it in a bold critique of post-Deleuzean materialism, as mentioned previously), the very constant production of surplus is plenty antagonistic, and it is this complication of a conative differential conception of the subject, nature and the body that makes life move 'forward'. This mode of continuity is also necessarily singular and creative as it will not repeat in negativity but transform in rupture. The chaotic rupture Guattari attributes to what is beyond language can be traced back to the experience of anxiety at the same time as it also informs the contemporary debate around a 'preservation' of sexual difference as an antidote to neoliberal capitalism. In very simple terms, a cartography of this logic could be mapped as such: it is only by 'going on' existing and living that the difference between the different attributes of substance is accumulated as a surplus. Surplus is this chaotic 'libidinal energy' that Freud observed as trying to find escape, in order to affect and be affected by other bodies, to move and in its detours is experienced as anxiety; it is the anxiety in the centre of Lacan's Borromean Knot, akin to a Real that is not entirely attached to the Symbolic.

In this sense, it is not simply or solely sexual difference as 'structuring' of the subject that can guarantee singularity—the route, as mentioned before, Zupančič' defends in *What is Sex?* (2017) for a critique of gender and queer theories which she sees as harnessed in the Imaginary. There is something of the order of the affective (affecting and affected) body, as it is experienced, that is excessive. This surplus generated in the difference between the full-void, phantasmatic, 'vibrating body' and 'consciousness' as such that reveals singularity and creativity in subjectivity is what is present in anxiety and, thus, fruitful to a non-Oedipal reading of Freud and Lacan. Anxiety, as an affect of rupture, brings up a body in flux, open to actualisations that are not bound to thought or symbolisation, thus a marker of a 'full-void, affective vibrating body', as inspired by Lygia Clark. Anxiety, in Freud's pre-1920s texts, cannot be subsumed in words, or interpretation and meaning. Anxiety, in this sense, is 'meaningless' but it is transformative as it insists and pushes the libidinal energy that is 'Life' onto the materiality of the body. This chaotic rupture, in its overwhelming presence, resonates what is described by 'attacks' of anxiety, or anxiety with all its deafening loud volume. At the same time, Lacan's 'lalangue', this poetic enjoyment of the order of the body, this unique, singular, inventive mode of speaking is also part of such 'chaos'. In this light, anxiety marks a territory of tension, this threshold between the relation to the Law (and by extension the patriarchal arrangement) and all that exists beyond it, the chaos that is in flux through the body and cannot be captured by language or words.

## Chaos, Vibration and the Clinic

Why insist on psychoanalysis, if it reproduces exactly what Clark moved beyond, namely, the Plane? Because not only can psychoanalysis denounce patriarchy by describing its operations and effects (Mitchell, 1974), but it may stop prescribing it, as long as it turns more chaotic, and less 'dividualising'. Following the trail of Clark, we can find clues for destabilising problematic anchors of psy-care practices, which limit the clinical treatment of rupture into an Oedipalised frame. More precisely, the 'full-void' of Clark's vibrational body proposes a subjective creation that starts from where there is no subject: in the void, there is fullness. It dismantles the necessity of subjective reproduction in accordance with the cultural echoes passed on by the colonial and patriarchal Symbolic as structured by the Phallic Law that is so pervasive in psy-practices.

Affect, symptom, noise and vibration. A body speaking in the world and an ecology that allows some sort of radical, resisting and transformative poietic existence is what I see in Lygia Clark's series *Structuring of the Self*. Her work invites us to Spinoza, whose "conative bodies are also associative or (one could even say) social bodies, in the sense that each is, by its very nature as a body, continuously affecting and being affected by other bodies" (Bennet, 2010, p. 21). This ontology thus proposes that we share the same substance which is in the world in different and differential modalities—akin to entangled 'differences without separability', as the epistemological and political turn proposed by Ferreira da Silva (2016). In sharp contrast to the negativity of desire (not to mention its connection with a 'need' and 'demand' that subscribe it to the phallic function in Lacan's early teachings), what moves our lives is not a repetition of negativity, but an affirmative tendency to produce difference anchored in this 'surplus' that is an excess of the order of experience that vibrates chaotically and creatively the 'full-void'. In other words, Clark's 'full-void' beyond the Plane operates as a metaphor, or a poetical wording of an understanding of affect as differential. This nuance is the reason why her practice is also specifically fruitful to my project that aims at re-orienting the psychoanalytic clinic of anxiety. It enables me to think-with Braidotti's 'nomadic subjectivity' in the clinic of this affect that is, ultimately, an affect of rupture, and thus being, claims space beyond a psychoanalytic clinic grounded on interpretation and its Oedipal foundations.

Guided by Clark's chaotic vibration—her full-void beyond the Plane; her sensations of the unconscious—we can think through what happens to the 'body in/of the world' and to the 'world with/of bodies' through the potency of a subjective full/void that vibrates independently from any Other. Here, the *sinthôme* Patricia Gherovici (2017) rescued in Lacan as a queer solution is expanded into collectivity—instead of working out one's excesses alone, Clark teaches us that what is beyond the Plane needs to be mobilised together, in *co-poiesis*. This collective nature of affect is exactly where we travel to in the foundations of the concept of 'vibration' in Deleuze and Guattari and take it with us to the clinic. Thinking-with Lygia Clark in alliance with Deleuze, Guattari, Braidotti, Rolnik and Spinoza has taken us to the fullness of the frontier, the novelty of chaos: In chaos we avoid the total reign of language and identity as well as materialist biological reductionism of experience. We meet chaos in the frontier of the vibrating 'full-void' of bodies.

## References

Allen, A. (2015). Are We Driven? Critical Theory and Psychoanalysis Reconsidered. *Critical Horizons, 4*(16), 311–328.

Baraitser, L. (2010). On Reading Transpositions: A Response to Rosi Braidotti's "Transpositions: On Nomadic Ethics". *Subjectivity, 3*, 125–130.

Benjamin, J. (1998). *Shadow of the Other – Intersubjectivity and Gender in Psychoanalysis*. Routledge.

Bennet, J. (2010). *Vibrant Matter: A Political Ecology of Things*. Duke University Press.

Berardi, F. (2015). *And. Phenomenology of the End*. Semiotext(e).

Berardi, F. (2018). *Breathing: Chaos and Poetry*. Semiotext(e).

Braidotti, R. (2006). *Transpositions: On Nomadic Ethics*. Polity Press.

Braidotti, R. (2011). *Nomadic Theory. The Portable Rosi Braidotti*. Columbia University Press.

Braidotti, R. (2017). *Per Una Politica Affermativa*. Mimesis Edizioni.

Butler, J. (1997). *The Psychic Life of Power: Theories in Subjection*. Stanford University Press.

Chiesa, L. (2016). *The Not-Two Logic and God in Lacan*. MIT Press.
Cigarini, L. (1995). *La Politica del Desiderio*. Pratiche.
Colebrook, C. (2000). *Deleuze and Feminist Theory*. Edinburgh University Press.
Curley, E. (1994). *A Spinoza Reader. The Ethics and Other works. Benedict de Spinoza* (E. Curley, Ed. and Trans.). Princeton University Press.
Deleuze, G., & Guattari, F. (1983). *Anti-Oedipus – Capitalism and Schizophrenia*. University of Minnesota Press.
Deleuze, G., & Guattari, F. (1987). *A Thousand Plateaus – Capitalism and Schizophrenia*. University of Minnesota Press.
Ettinger, B. (2006). *The Matrixial Borderspace*. University of Minnesota Press.
Ettinger, B. (2019). Beyond the Death-Drive, Beyond the Life-Drive: Being-toward-Birthing with Being-toward-Birth; Copoiesis and the Matrixial Eros—Metafeminist Notes. In P. De Assis & P. Giudici (Eds.), *Aberrant Nuptials: Deleuze and Artistic Research*. Leuven University Press.
Federici, S. (2019). *Re-enchanting the World: Feminism and the Politics of the Commons*. PM Press/Kairos.
Federici, S. (2020). *Beyond the Periphery of the Skin: Rethinking, Remaking, and Reclaiming the Body in Contemporary Capitalism*. PM Press/Kairos.
Ferreira da Silva, D. (2016). On Difference Without Separability. Catalogue of the 32nd *São Paulo Art Biennial 'Incerteza Viva'*, pp. 57–65.
Fouque, A. (1995). *Il y a deux sexes: essais de féminologie. 1989–1995*. Gallimard.
Gatens, M., & Lloyd, G. (1999). *Collective Imaginings: Spinoza, Past and Present*. Routledge.
Gherovici, P. (2017). *Transgender Psychoanalysis: A Lacanian Perspective on Sexual Difference*. Routledge.
Grosz, E. (2007). Deleuze, Bergson and the Concept of Life. *Revue Internationale de Philosophie, 241*(3), 287–300.
Grosz, E. (2008). *Chaos, Territory, Art: Deleuze and the Framing of the Earth*. Columbia University Press.
Grosz, E. (2017). *The Incorporeal: Ontology, Ethics, and the Limits of Materialism*. Columbia University Press.
Guattari, F. (1989). *Schizoanalytic Cartographies*. Bloomsbury.
Guattari, F. (1995a). *Chaosmosis. An Ethico-aesthetic Paradigm*. Indiana University Press.
Guattari, F. (1995b). *The Machinic Unconscious: Essays in Schizoanalysis*. Semiotext (e).
Guattari, F. (2000). *The Three Ecologies*. The Athlone Press.
Guattari, F. (2006). *Anti-Oedipus Papers*. Semiotext(e).
Guattari, F. (2009). *Chaosophy: Texts and Interviews 1972 1977*. Semiotext(e).

Guattari, F. (2015). *Psychoanalysis and Transversality: Texts and Interviews 1955-1971*. Semiotext (e).
Guattari, F., & Rolnik, S. (2007). *Molecular Revolution in Brazil*. Semiotext(e).
Haraway, D. (2016). *Staying with the Trouble: Making Kin in the Chthulucene*. Duke University Press.
Khanna, R. (2003). *Dark Continents: Psychoanalysis and Colonialism, Post-Contemporary Interventions*. Duke University Press.
Kordela, K. (2007). *Surplus: Spinoza, Lacan*. SUNY Press.
Lacan, J. (1993). *The Psychoses. The Seminar of Jacques Lacan Book III, 1955-1956*. Routledge.
Miller, J.A. (2003). 'Lacan's Later Teaching'. Lacanian Ink . Vol.21 Spring.2003. [Online] http://www.lacan.com/frameXXI2.htm
Mitchell, J. (1974). *Psychoanalysis and Feminism*. Patheon.
Mitchell, J. (1982). Introduction 1. In J. Mitchell & J. Rose (Eds.), *Feminine Sexuality – Jacques Lacan and the école freudienne*. Norton-Pantheon.
Preciado, P. B. (2020). *Je suis um Monstre qui vous parle. Rapport pour une academie de psychanalystes*. Bernard Grasset.
Rolnik, S. (1989). *Cartografia Sentimental. Transformações contemporâneas do desejo*. Estação Liberdade.
Rolnik, S. (2000, April 30). O corpo vibrátil de Lygia Clark. *Folha de Sao Paulo* [Online]. https://www1.folha.uol.com.br/fsp/mais/fs3004200006.htm
Rolnik, S. (2015). Beyond the Colonial Unconscious. *Art and Education* [Online]. https://www.artandeducation.net/classroom/video/66076/suely-rolnik-beyond-colonial-unconscious
Rolnik, S. (2019). *Esferas da Insurreição: notas para uma vida não cafetinada*. n-1.
Roudinesco, E. (2020, June 12). Je suis un monstre qui vous parle »: la « psychanalyse mutante » de Paul B. Preciado. *Le Monde* [Online]. https://www.lemonde.fr/livres/article/2020/06/12/je-suis-un-monstre-qui-vous-parle-la-psychanalyse-mutante-de-paul-b-preciado_6042598_3260.html
Sabsay, L. (2016). *The Political Imaginary of Sexual Freedom Subjectivity and Power in the New Sexual Democratic Turn*. Palgrave.
Sauvagnargues, A. (2016). *Artmachines: Deleuze, Guattari, Simondon*. Edinburgh University Press.
Schuster, A. (2016). *The trouble with pleasure. Deleuze and Psychoanalysis*. The MIT Press.
Soler, C. (2014). *Lacanian Affects: The Function of Affect in Lacan's Work*. Routledge.
Tuhkanen, M. (2009). Performativity and Becoming. *Cultural Critique, 72*, 1–35.
Watson, J. (2009). *Guattari's Diagrammatic Thought Writing Between Lacan and Deleuze*. Continuum.

Williams, A., & Srnicek, N. (2013, May 14). #ACCELERATE MANIFESTO for an Accelerationist Politics. *Critical Legal Thinking* [Online]. https://criticallegalthinking.com/2013/05/14/accelerate-manifesto-for-an-accelerationist-politics/

Zamboni, C. (2019). La pratica dell'inconscio. Un ponte tra "Psychanalyse et Politique", Antoinette Fouque e il pensiero femminista italiano. *Per Amore del Mondo*, Vol. 16 [Online]. http://www.diotimafilosofe.it/wp-content/uploads/2019/11/Zamboni_Inconscio-tra-Fouque-e-Cigarini-Parigi-2016-1.pdf

Žižek, S. (1992). *Enjoy Your Symptom!* Routledge.

Žižek, S. (2004). *Organs Without Bodies: On Deleuze and Consequences*. Routledge.

Žižek, S. (2010). *Interrogating the Real*. Continuum.

Žižek, S. (2016, August 1). The Sexual is Political. *The Philosophical Salon* [Online]. http://thephilosophicalsalon.com/the-sexual-is-political

Zupančič, A. (2017). *What Is Sex?* MIT Press.

Zupančič, A. (2019, October 7). On Sex Without Identity: Feminist Politics and Sexual Difference. *Los Angeles Review of Books* [Online]. https://lareviewofbooks.org/article/sex-without-identity-feminist-politics-sexual-difference/

# 8

# The Trail of Vibration

After mapping 'vibrational moments' in both Freud and Lacan as possible entries into 'becomings' versus a dividualising 'being' as the clinical paradigm of anxiety, we will dive deeper into the concept of vibration and its genealogy in the work of Deleuze and Guattari. We will cross their theories of affect and subjectivity in order to find grounds for a 'vibrational clinic'. Building on the *co-poietic* method of the artist Lygia Clark in her later works, and especially *Structuring of the Self* series, I will map a possible model of clinical assemblage in Guattari's 'transversal' take on anxiety. The difficulty and at times contradictions of Deleuze and Guattari's varied and rich work and their Anti-Oedipal approach anchor our alliance with Lygia Clark: here as a horizon-beyond a view of anxiety that is reduced to an abyss-within (or an enigma of the body of the order of sexuality as organised under the phallic paradigm).

Deleuze and Guattari have offered important critiques of psychoanalysis in the second half of the twentieth century as part of their philosophical, political and clinical enterprise. Together and separately, they have questioned the model of repression and negative repetition in symptoms, the centrality of a subjective organisation structured under the Oedipal model and the form of an 'ego', as well as the clinical relationship framework based on a dual transference that, to them, "modelled itself after the



A. C. Minozzo, *Anxiety as Vibration*, Studies in the Psychosocial,
https://doi.org/10.1007/978-3-031-62856-6_8

contractual relationship of the most traditional bourgeois medicine: the feigned exclusion of a third party; the hypocritical role of money, to which psychoanalysis brought farcical new justifications" (Deleuze & Guattari, 1983, p. 84). The psychoanalytic frame perpetuated and practiced by the establishment also relied on "the pretended time limitation that contradicts itself by reproducing a debt to infinity, by feeding an inexhaustible transference, and by always nursing new 'conflicts'" (Deleuze & Guattari, 1983, p. 84). To use Deleuze's (1992) own word, psychoanalysis wished to propose a life in touch with the unconscious but remained 'dividualising' or alienating and modulating subjectivity through a stiff ideological mechanism and onto-epistemic foundation.

Their work has been influential in the field of critical theories, new philosophical interventions and the arts. However, within the clinical landscape (from psychoanalytic training programmes to institutional practices in mental health care), their concepts have been largely ignored or swiftly brushed off in defensive accusations of mis-reading Freud and Lacan—for example, in their famous critique to the psychoanalytic privileging of a neurotic subject (David-Menard, 2014). Save for a very limited array of attempts to question the potentialities of the body, affect and the limits of language as a tool of interpretation and punctuation (Suely Rolnik and Monique David-Menard being two important examples, in Latin America and in Europe), their 'schizoanalysis' is mostly discussed in theoretical works that dispute the concept of 'desire' (Schuster, 2016) and the discrepancies between the philosophical approaches of Hegel and Spinoza (Moder, 2017). In this cartographic exercise, I do not wish to pursue an in-depth investigation on the possibilities of 'correcting' psychoanalysis with Deleuze and Guattari's ideas. Neither do I wish to call in a psychoanalytic 'authority' over Deleuze and Guattari's writings (Felman, 1982), which would be to denounce their naiveté facing 'real' suffering or even their theoretical alliance to a kind of postmodern neoliberal affirmation without necessary antagonism (Žižek, 2010, 2017). Rather, my aim is to find in their theory and practice, respectively, points that can illuminate the knots on Freudian-Lacanian conceptions of anxiety in an attempt to establish a common ground between these two theoretical approaches and clinical practices that bring about an eco-feminist ethics in light of the contemporary psychosocial context—namely, the possibilities for interdependence rather than domination as the matrix of relation to others instead of with the Other—which I do so by following Rosi Braidotti (1994, 2006a, 2006b, 2011, 2013, 2017, 2019).[1] My way into this complex endeavour is via the formulation of the concept of 'anxiety as vibration' and the guiding compass is the search for affirmative and differential nuances in the psychosomatic (or psychic and somatic) experience of the affect of anxiety. Informed by the clinical and conceptual 'dividualisations' reproduced in psychoanalysis and by the potency of its critique in Lygia Clark's 'full-void' vibrational body, in what follows, I trace the 'trail' of vibration in Deleuze and Guattari's work in relation to affect, possibility and the friction between 'being' and 'becomings', as a ground that moves the rupture of the affect of anxiety from an abyss-within into a horizon-beyond.

## Vibration between Ontology and Ethics

Deleuze's ontology is centred on difference. His thinking is heavily influenced by his original reading of Nietzsche, Bergson and Spinoza, as well as Leibniz and Simondon, all of whom had been extremely unfashionable during the 1950s and 1960s in France, where the 'three Hs' (Hegel, Heidegger and Husserl) reigned in Philosophy departments, according to Dosse (2010). Deleuze takes from Spinoza the idea that an ontology that works against the notion of the transcendent in favour of immanence (in general terms, accepting that there is just one substance, God and nature being this same substance) is the basis of an ethics. It is with shy irony that Deleuze points out in his course on Spinoza, delivered in Vincennes, that Spinoza did not call his seventeenth century monograph 'Ontology', rather, he named it his 'Ethics'. In what touches Deleuze's critique of psychoanalysis, especially Lacanian psychoanalysis and the absorption of

[1] By holding on to vibration, I am also stressing the unconscious factor of such 'commons', agreeing with and complementing Stacey Alaimo's posthumanist concept of transcorporeality. Alaimo (2014) proposes that "we are entangled with multiple material agencies, flows and processes that connect human bodies, animal bodies, ecosystems, technologies, and the wider world. As the material self cannot be disentangled from networks that are simultaneously environmental, economic, political, cultural, scientific, technological, and substantial, what was once the ostensibly bounded human subject finds herself in a swirling landscape of uncertainty where practices and actions that were once not even remotely ethical or political matters suddenly become so" (Alaimo, 2014, p. 17).

the Freudian concepts of the resolution of the Oedipus Complex into a structuralist model, this detail assumes particular relevance.

To start the examination of the concept of vibration, we could consider this ethical and ontological dispute as follows. Culturally specific, and perhaps culturally hegemonic, language/Symbolic structures take the transcendental 'One' (the phallic father inscribed in the Oedipal myth) as a necessity or even a 'given fact' in 'reality', informing thus several aspects of our subjective inscription, such as the potential and possibilities for life under or outside the 'Law'. In this sense, here we situate Lacan's Other and the Law-of-the-Father as anchors of the Symbolic register and towards which a subjective structure is directed, revealing a particular inscription of transcendentalism in Lacan—seeing that the fundamental structuring of the subject relies on preconditions external to it, a definition of 'transcendental' offered by Jean Wahl (1944 [2016]).[2] Neurosis, perversion or psychosis are then seen as the only possible outcomes of this necessary relation. Under the ethical and ontological approach proposed by Deleuze and by Guattari, there is something more primordial to the 'subject' as framed in 'culture' as such that pertains to the relation of the unique 'substance' that appears in the world only in different intensities, as Spinoza posits in his *Ethics*. These intensities, in Spinoza, and as rescued by Deleuze in his first book on the Dutch philosopher from 1968 (*Spinoza et le problème de l'expression)*, the second from 1981 (*Spinoza—Philosophie pratique*) and the Vincennes lectures, compose what is called 'affect'. An interesting definition of affect from Deleuze's lecture in Vincennes on the 24th of January 1978 reads: "Every mode of thought insofar as it is non-representational will be termed affect" (Deleuze, 1978).[3] This relation between affect and thought and their logical, intrinsic and extrinsic differences is unpacked in this particular lecture of his *Sur Spinoza* course, a crucial difference, as we will see in what follows. Not only the non-representability of affect, but its collectivity, the point that it does not feature in the Symbolic and the connection it holds with the body are the basis for the 'vibrating' ability of such intensities that

[2] In *Human Existence and Transcendence* (1944) Jean Wahl defines the transcendent as in one side what transcends the human (the divine in religious terms) and in another side the movement of the human reaching beyond itself.

[3] My translation of the French original "*on appellera affect tout mode de pensée qui ne représente rien*".

cross bodies, which constantly affect each other. Affect, in this model, also resists the need for a transcendental 'third' or 'power' anchoring it, it does not need an 'Other' with capital 'O'.[4] Affect is, for Spinoza, "the power to affect and be affected" (Massumi, 2015, p. ix), rather than a 'substance' or ethereal potion travelling through bodies like electricity as other affect theorists will mistakenly interpret.[5] Affect, for Deleuze, is more of an ethical capacity beyond universal frames of representation than an 'electric current' behaving like a contaminating virus across bodies.

In *Francis Bacon: The Logic of Sensation*, first published in 1981, Deleuze famously affirms that "sensation is vibration" (Deleuze, 2003, p. 45). In this piece, Deleuze writes about how Bacon was trying to paint 'sensations' rather than figurative representations when painting bodies. I find this a useful analogy to approach this question of language and of the 'representability' of things, taking us on a journey to think how words are charged with affect but also to meet, in clear psychoanalytic terms, the limits of identification (Imaginary identification being the frame of anxiety, as per Lacan in Seminar X; and it is based on the principle of 'Sameness' grounded over the idea of the 'One', as proposed by Braidotti, 2006a). Deleuze's work on sensation presents us with a view of a body that is 'beyond' language, is vibrating, and is also in movement as it affects and is affected by other bodies. We must, however, be careful to see in this non-representability an ethical stance rather than a mystical 'feeling', 'emotion', 'electric current' or a production of the body beyond words that gets transmitted through bodies. Honing into the matter of affect and exploring this ethical ontological project, started by Deleuze and carried on through his encounter with Félix Guattari and scholars influenced by them since, will take us to a questioning of what is representable according to Freud and Lacan and how have both psychoanalytic models accounted for what is not. The Lacanian Real, which is

---

[4] Whilst I reference Brian Massumi, I am not necessarily aligning myself with his thought, once it is relevant to mention that feminist theories of affect such as that of Sara Ahmed (2004) or Emily Martin (2013) have found his work to be problematic for it ignores the social sphere completely. Ahmed's (2004) claim for emotion and affect to be grounded in relationality is not too dissimilar in its ethics to what Guattari goes on to elaborate in his actual clinical practice of transversality.

[5] Silvan Tomkins' interpretation of Deleuze would lead into Paul Ekman's extremely controversial theories of affect and feelings beyond cognition which, not surprisingly, led him to collaborate with the CIA and the FBI (Tomkins & Smith, 1995).

carefully sculpted through the decades of his teachings, is the central contrast with the model of 'sensation' that we find in Deleuze. As we will rescue, across their work and very clearly in Guattari's sole writings, the matter of 'representability' versus 'non-representability' is diffracted further into the notion of 'polyvocity' (Genosko, 2002) that is central to what I identify here as Guattari's theory of anxiety.

A longer definition of 'affect' in Deleuze's reading of Spinoza invites us to consider 'variation' and 'possibility' as elements of affect that resonate a further excursion into Deleuze and Guattari's notion of 'vibration'. Deleuze's lesson on Spinoza in Vincennes in late January 1978 elicits the ethical and 'relational' character of affect in its detailed difference from an 'idea/thought'. Relational here, is not as a relation between similar 'objects', in a traditional psychoanalytic sense as per the British Tradition, for example, but of all 'bodies', thus nature as 'all there is', following Spinoza. Deleuze unpacks affect, first saying that we can differentiate an 'idea' and an affect by considering that an idea is a mode of thought that represents something, whilst an affect is a mode of thought that represents nothing. This is a technical and nominal differentiation based on 'external and extrinsic' factors. The second layer of this differentiation Deleuze reads in Spinoza is more complicated: whilst an idea has an intrinsic reality, "affect is the continuous variation or the passage from one degree of reality to another" (Deleuze, January 24, 1978).[6] Beyond the nominal difference, we have now also a 'real difference', which opens up the 'possibilities' of a thing and not just its description. Affect, he continues, "it is the continuous variation of the force of existing of anyone" (Deleuze, January 24, 1978).[7] The force of existing, as Spinoza outlines in his ethics, is named 'conatus'; thus, affect would be this continuous variation of conatus. He completes: "insofar as this variation is determined by the ideas one has" (Deleuze, January 24, 1978).[8] This 'determination' of affect by ideas and yet the irreducibility of affect to ideas is the conundrum Deleuze explores in the differentiation of Spinoza's terms

[6] My translation of French original: "*l'affect, c'est la variation continue ou le passage d'un degré de réalité à un autre*".

[7] My translation of French original: "*c'est donc la variation continue de la force d'exister de quelqu'un*".

[8] My translation of French original: "*en tant que cette variation est déterminée par les idées qu'il a*".

'affectio' and 'affectus', Latin terms he claims were all mistranslated from the Ethics as 'affect', but which still carry a difference, and one interesting to psychoanalysis. Affectus would be 'affect', and what we have described so far, whilst 'affectio' is 'affection', defined as the 'mixing' (*mélange*) of bodies and the changes or consequences that entail the effects over the nature of these bodies. Being in the world and the *mélange* of bodies resonate—*affectio*—on ideas (representational), which, in their turn, determine *affectus, the* non-representational kinds of thoughts. Affect, thus, seems to be not just transindividual but collective or 'collaborative' in essence, an ethical disposition.

To summarise and clarify, Deleuze's take on Spinoza's theory of affect has it that affect is not of the order of representation, it escapes it; affect has to do with the variations of one's force of existing; and these variations will be determined by the effects of our encounter with other bodies—determined, not reduced to, neither represented by—which can only be grasped by our ideas of the consequences of such encounters (e.g. the sun on my skin, meeting someone on the street, etc.). The difficulty of these abstract lectures may be why Deleuze's (as well as Guattarri's) ideas have been so misinterpreted as it is easy to read affect as something quite 'magical' and beyond words that happens when we meet others in the world. Deleuze here reminds us of another layer of Spinoza's oeuvre that is essential to keep in mind: his view of the limitations of our repertoire of 'ideas', our experience of grasping reality through ideas one after another vis-à-vis the passages of one degree of reality to another, which is the character of affect, as we have just seen. Drawing on Spinoza's *Tractatus Theologico-Politicus* (published posthumously in 1677), Deleuze points out that to him we are fabricated as spiritual automatons, with ideas succeeding one another all the time in us, determining our potentiality of acting or our force of existing in a continuous line. Spinoza sees the 'soul' as a machine of ideas, immanent and self-determined. Catherine Malabou (2016) in fact adds to the Deleuzean reading of the *Ethics,* by arguing that Spinoza's *Treatise* functions between the duality of transcendence and immanence, proposing a theory of the origin of the Symbolic (in the Spinozean monist version of God/the sacred) with no reference outside of itself. Here we reach a paradox in relation to psychoanalysis, for, if anything, words and ideas are in Lacan necessarily crossed by the field of the Other, or Symbolically arranged, and a rupture in this crossing would indicate the side of psychosis. What Deleuze draws from Spinoza and what goes on to influence so much of his work with Guattari and the thinkers influenced by them to present day (such as Rolnik and Braidotti, as I we engage with closely across this cartography of anxiety)—the notion of desire as immanent and of affect as an excess to representation that travels in encounters—disputes the central Structuralist and Post-Structuralist tenets of Lacanian psychoanalysis that see in a Symbolic arrangement the net in which subjectivity is constructed, either through meaning or gaps in meaning, nonetheless determined by symbolisation. Here, again, we find an interesting alignment with what I called Freud and Lacan's 'vibrational moments' as well as with Lygia Clark's vibrational 'full-void': there is scope for an immanent production of affect which does not cross or is not reduced by its relation to the Oedipal Other and the Symbolic as such. Rather, we find here sustenance for a view of the *sinthôme* as an articulation of the Real into novel Imaginaries—as Lacan (1975) proposes in his Seminar XXIII, being a creative solution that does not call for interpretation; rather, as Lygia Clark proposes and I hold onto here, calling for a communal, collective construction, a *co-poiesis*.

Deleuze and Guattari work through this ethical-ontological muddle throughout their lives. In what concerns psychoanalysis their quest could be translated, as I read it, in simple terms, by asking "how much of me is left beyond representational ideas?"; "what are the qualities of what is left?"; and "can we think of an ethical and political landscape of these excesses?". In *Anti-Oedipus* and *A Thousand Plateaus* they try, in more direct psychoanalytic terms, to meditate through libido, the Real, the drive, the body and language. They go beyond the sources that founded psychoanalysis and of psychoanalysis itself to think through these ethical possibilities, contextualising the psychoanalytic discourse as pertaining to a context of capitalism and repression, binarism and patriarchy. An ethical capacity beyond the dualism of representation would open the way for the invention of new worlds and novel forms of living—or a sprout/seedling of the world that lives in us, 'gérmens de mundo' (Rolnik, 2019), an opening of the 'paradoxical body' (Gil, 1998) would be mobilised in this affective turn. Such *co-poietic* processes of reinvention would start with the body (in affects, symptoms, ruptures) and create new words and worlds, invoking a collectivity without crossing the field of the Other as a subordinate. In other words, it is from affects that 'being' can be extended into 'becomings'.

For Brian Massumi, "the concept of affect is politically oriented from the get go" (Massumi, 2015, p. viii). Massumi is part of a generation of theorists dedicated to 'affect', an early-2000s theoretical trend known as the 'affective turn', which counts with diverse names such as Rosi Braidotti, Eve Kosofsky Sedgwick, Silvan Tomkins and Elizabeth Grosz. Ideas proposing that affects vibrate, especially in relation to the body, which is an archaic, pre-linguistic, transindividual body, and of the level of a 'body knowledge' (Massumi, 2015, p. 210), are relevant to my delineation of 'anxiety as vibration', and require that we go through Deleuze and Guattari's work in more detail, stressing Guattari's realm of 'chaos' rather than the paradigm of a 'repository' as Massumi (2015) seems to propose. The confusion and the danger of thinking of what is not of the order of representation—or what is beyond the Plane, in Clark's words—and that leaves traces on the body as a kind of 'magical substance' have been pointed out by several critics of the affect theorists for the risk of a lack of ethical possibilities when focusing on states beyond cognition/consciousness (Hemmings, 2005; Leys, 2017). We could think of this as simply the ethical possibilities of the unconscious, and, more precisely, as the ethical possibilities of the 'body whilst unconscious trace', much as contemporary Lacanians work with the idea that the speaking-body is the twenty-first century unconscious (Miller, 2014), or the ethics of the Real (Brousse, 2007). I take this question as central to the psychopolitics of the clinic, once it is necessary to account for the process of 'dividualisation' and estrangement from anxiety. Being able to mobilise possibilities that further the subject reduced to a dividual would be the ethical and political necessity of a contemporary 'couch revolution' that is truly faithful to Freud's project in light of contemporary epistemological demands (Preciado, 2020)—namely, ecological, social, political changes and urgencies that challenge the epistemology of alienation found in the psychoanalytic dividualising Oedipal abyss-within.

Deleuze's philosophical project, which starts with the 1953 publication of *Empirisme et subjectivité: Essai sur la nature humaine selon Hume* and ends with the 1993 publication of *Critique et Clinique*, can be understood in the context of his engagement with a particular version of empiricism and a critique of transcendentalism in philosophy, from which he will thus enter the field of psychoanalysis along the way, alone and with Félix Guattari. For Deleuze and Guattari in *What is Philosophy*, published in English in 1994, philosophy was an empirical project insofar as it involved 'conceptual creations'. They write: "philosophy is the art of forming, inventing, and fabricating concepts" (Deleuze & Guattari, 1994, p. 2) and this creation is done without appeal to a transcendental illusion. Deleuze writes in the preface to the English edition of *Dialogues* that he always considered himself to be an empiricist thinker, by which he means he is a 'pluralist'. In this rich short introduction to his dialogue with Claire Parnet, he explains that, for him at least, empiricism involved accounting for multiplicity without resorting to a universal or eternal in order to explain the "conditions under which something new is produced (creativeness)" (Deleuze & Parnet, 1987, p. vii), without abstracting the totalities of the One, the Whole or the Subject, rationalist traps that, as he sees it, psychoanalysis has fallen into. Empiricism, or his philosophical endeavour, starts by "analysing the states of things, in such a way that non-pre-existent concepts can be extracted from them. States of things are neither unities nor totalities, but *multiplicities*" (Deleuze & Parnet, 1987, p. vii). This idea of multiplicity is important to comprehend; it:

> Designates a set of lines or dimensions which are irreducible to one another. Every 'thing' is made up in this way. Of course a multiplicity includes focuses of unification, centres of totalization, points of subjectivation, but as factors which can prevent its growth and stop its lines.[…] In a multiplicity what counts are not the terms or the elements, but what there is 'between', the between, as set of relations which are not separable from each other. Every multiplicity grows from the middle, like the blade of grass or the rhizome. We constantly oppose the rhizome to the tree, like two conceptions and even two very different ways of thinking. (Deleuze & Parnet, 1987, pp. vii–viii)

Psychoanalysis, under this logic, is at first 'empiricist' enough, but it surrenders to the rationalist (and typically modern, colonial and patriarchal) illusion of totalities and loses its political potency. Freud, for

Deleuze, at first sees the multiplicities in the polymorphous perversion of the "skin as a collection of pores, the slipper, the field of stitches" (Deleuze & Parnet, 1987, p. viii), yet he "constantly fell back on the calmer vision of a neurotic unconscious which plays with eternal abstractions" (Deleuze & Parnet, 1987, p. viii). Klein, "even Melanie Klein" he writes, granting her special respect, also succumbs to the same logic for her "partial objects still refer to a unity, even if it is lost, to a totality, even if it is to come, to a subject, even if it is split" (Deleuze & Parnet, 1987, p. ix). What Deleuze strives with his philosophical project, and the collaboration with Guattari, is to create concepts that engage with multiplicity, as a means to imagine novel possibilities of being. He writes: "It seemed to us [him and Guattari] that politics is at stake as well and that in a social field rhizome spread out everywhere under the arborescent apparatuses" (Deleuze & Parnet, 1987, p. ix). The conditions for the emergence of such novelty is the kernel of a possible "couch revolution", that a feminist and Deleuzian-Guattarian critique of psychoanalysis calls for (Preciado, 2018).

The way Deleuze starts engaging with such multiplicities is by his reading, interpretation and creation of concepts from the works of Spinoza and Bergson (Deleuze & Guattari, 1994), mainly, as they allow him to consider a 'radical empiricism' through the idea of a 'plane of immanence'. Such a plane, Deleuze and Guattari write, "does not present a flux of the lived that is immanent to a subject and individualised in that which belongs to a self. It presents only events, that is, possible worlds as concepts, and other people as expressions of possible worlds or conceptual personae" (Deleuze & Guattari, 1994, pp. 47–48). This 'plane of immanence' is, as they write, "surrounded by illusions" (Deleuze & Guattari, 1994, p. 49): the illusion of transcendence, the illusion of universals, the illusion of the eternal and the illusion of discursiveness (Deleuze & Guattari, 1994). These illusions lock possibilities and erase multiplicity condemning it into a relation to a referential and transcendental One (interestingly resonating Lygia Clark's *Nostalgia of the Body* essay). Here we can see their resistance to tracing concepts by a traditional genealogy that stays firmly closed to a tradition of history of philosophy, as the historical is a taming of the potentiality of multiplicity and invention of new modes of being—which they call an 'event'. They write:

> Philosophy cannot be reduced to its own history, because it continually wrests itself from this history in order to create new concepts that fall back into history but do not come from it. How could something come from history? Without history, becoming would remain indeterminate and unconditioned, but becoming is not historical. Psychosocial types belong to history, but conceptual personae belong to becoming. (Deleuze &Guattari, 1994, p. 96)

In this sense, we cannot reduce an ontology (conceptual personae) to history as we will then be simply describing what exists under the agreed universal conditions—or illusions—rather than opening up possibilities of the order of the plane of immanence. In other words, "psychosocial types are historical, but conceptual personae are events" (Deleuze & Guattari, 1994, p. 110). The question of their relation to the plane of immanence and a critique to the transcendental takes us back to the question of 'affect' and how affects cannot be reduced to 'opinions' or pre-arranged set-ups; rather, they should be allowed to be recombined, coupled, to vibrate and to 'create' or 'become'. Discussing literature, art and psychoanalysis, they point at the limiting of 'opinion' or 'ideas' over affects, of imposing 'knowledge' over an affect and thus classifying it and mapping preconditioned futures to such affective possibilities and 'becomings'.

Psychoanalysis, philosophy, literature and art should engage with such immanence instead of being limited to the transcendental 'tree' of universal referential conditions such as the 'Other' and the 'Law'. Psychoanalysis should then, according to this logic, account for the possibility of vibrations—of affect recombination, creation and a political ontology that is in tune with contemporary epistemological, ecological and political demands that stem off the epistemology of alienation and the logic domination—rather than map and reproduce psychosocial historical subjects. With this motivation in mind, I embark on a search for vibration.

In order to dive fully into what Deleuze and Guattari mean by 'vibration', and to prepare the ground to my thinking of 'anxiety as vibration', I follow below with a cartographic genealogy of the concept of vibration, discussing how it is crucial to the understanding of notion of 'sensation' and of 'affect' within this tradition of thinking. My reading method is cartographic-rhizomatic, meaning that I follow the word 'vibration' across key texts from Deleuze and Guattari, opening up into their conceptualisations of the body, affect and an ontology in the dynamic genesis of language and its relation to the limits of the Symbolic (not to forget, a Symbolic that is, for them, Oedipally framed and thus charged with the Eurocentric colonialist patriarchal and capitalist subjective mode within the epistemology of alienation and domination), pausing and digressing as 'vibration' leads.

## The Trail of Vibration

When discussing the oeuvre of Bergson, who will, along with Spinoza, prove to be a fundamental influence in Deleuze and Guattari's ontological model, in the book *Bergsonism*, first published in 1966 in French, Deleuze delineates the materialist monism of Bergson in relation to perception, time (duration) and what extends 'beyond us' or our experience beyond the individual as per Bergson's monograph *Matter and Memory*. He writes:

> At each instant, our perception contracts "an incalculable multitude of rememorized elements"; at each instant, our present infinitely contracts our past: "The two terms which had been separated to begin with cohere closely together... *What, in fact, is a sensation? It is the operation of contracting trillions of vibrations onto a receptive surface* [my emphasis]. Quality emerges from this, quality that is nothing other than contracted quantity". (Deleuze, 1991, p. 74)

Perception and memory, or recollection, become 'one' in Bergson under this energetic metaphor of quantity of vibrations from the 'outside', or beyond the body, into a sensation where it can turn into a 'quality', in what I read to be similar to what in Spinoza and in Deleuze will be called affect. As Deleuze writes, "*Matter and Memory* recognizes intensities, degrees or vibrations in the qualities that we live as such outside ourselves and that, as such, belong to matter" (Deleuze, 1991, p. 92). According to Elizabeth Grosz (2007), Bergson's influence on Deleuze allows him to think not in terms of vitalism (even though Bergson speaks of an *élan vital*) that would presuppose finality or a total, rather in terms of life as a process, or affirmation since for Bergson "life assumes a continuous, never ceasing relation of change" (Grosz, 2007, p. 294). To think in terms of intensities that vibrate takes Deleuze away from other dominant modes of thinking about life and the body, moving away from organicism and from phenomenology once "each places the functional or experiencing body as a given rather than as the effect of processes of continual creation, movement or individuation" (Grosz, 2007, p. 289). For Grosz this ecological ontology that we see in Deleuze's collaboration with Guattari—and very clearly in Guattari's solo work such as *The Three Ecologies*, from 1989—can be traced to the influence of Bergson, since, as she writes it is *Bergsonism* that contributes with "an understanding of individuality as a kind of dynamic integrative absorption of an outside that is always too much, too large, to be ordered and contained within life alone, but which extends life beyond itself into the very reaches of the inorganic" (Grosz, 2007, pp. 288–289).

In *Difference and Repetition*, first published in French in 1968, Deleuze speaks to psychoanalysis very closely as he offers a unique reading of Freud's *Beyond the Pleasure Principle*. The question of primary repression and of the origins of the unconscious is tackled by invoking terms from philosophy and literature to think of 'habit', 'memory' and what is it that makes repetition repeat. Deleuze, already in this piece, forces a reading of repetition against the model of repression: "I do not repeat because I repress. I repress because I repeat, I forget because I repeat. I repress, because I can live certain things or certain experiences only in the mode of repetition. I am determined to repress whatever would prevent me from living them thus: in particular, the representation which mediates the lived by relating it to the form of a similar or identical object" (Deleuze, 1995, p. 18). Repetition is seen as a positivity, it is akin to a rupture, or a gap, that is central to the conflict of the drives (Eros and Thanatos, as he takes from Freud). Rather than being a characteristic of a 'glitch' of the conscious system, it entails difference or new qualities each time we repeat. In this book, on the first page, Deleuze uses the word *vibration* for the first time in relation to the unconscious. He does not develop this idea in the book at all, but the meaning it bears here, of a reverberation of a *conative* (in Spinoza's terms) character of the body, remains important. Deleuze writes: "To repeat is to behave in a certain manner, but in relation to something unique or singular which has no equal or equivalent. And perhaps this repetition at the level of external conduct echoes, for its own part, a more secret vibration which animates it, a more profound, internal repetition within the singular" (Deleuze, 1995, p. 1). The positive and differential unconscious emerges through the movement of the drive, it vibrates in repetition. If what is repressed, primarily, are not representations—as Deleuze puts it, 'presentations' are the material of the Freudian primary repression (Deleuze, 1995)—but what, as we can interpret, is not of the order of representation, therefore affect, then affects constitute the core of such 'founding' elements of the unconscious. In a way, this does not take us very far from Freud's theories of the drive as this encounter of psyche and soma—which is not all psy nor all soma, but a 'body' of a 'different order' that appears in the drive.

Deleuze follows this line of thought in *Logic of Sense*, published for the first time in the following year, 1969. One of the most interesting aspects of this piece, in what concerns this research, is his exposition and critique of the psychoanalytic theories of Melanie Klein. The drives and what 'moves' this encounter of psyche-soma in her theories of a fragmented body form his central arguments about language, or 'sense' as it is 'written over' the body. This book tackles a variety of philosophical and literary ideas to explore the genesis of 'sense' (and nonsense), arriving at the conditions of sense being, necessarily, outside of what is 'meant' by any proposition, "the expressed makes possible the expression" (Deleuze, 1990, p. 186). Meaning, thus, is transcendental and relates to what Lacan calls the Symbolic order, as we can interpret from this part of the book. The second part of the book is more attractive to readers less familiar with analytic philosophy and logic (resources strongly pulled together in the first part) as it will then explore the conditions of the genesis of language from a rather unique interpretation of Klein, sounds, expression and the body. Despite not speaking about 'vibration' directly in this book, Deleuze discusses intensities that cross the infant's body in fragmented and chaotic manners borrowing from Daniel Stern and Melanie Klein as well as Artaud, inaugurating his theorising of the 'Body without Organs' here.

In his account, infants are born into bodily noises, sounds and primary affects. These sounds from the 'depths' will be mobilised into language and the production of sense/nonsense thereafter. He writes: "When we say that the sound becomes independent, we mean to say that it ceases to be a specific quality attached to bodies, a noise or a cry, and that it begins to designate qualities, manifest bodies, and signify subjects or predicates" (Deleuze, 1990, p. 187). He is interested in the 'surface' that is produced as language happens, curious about the "depth-surface distinction [which] is, in every respect, primary in relation to the distinctions nature-convention, nature-custom, or nature-artifice" (Deleuze, 1990, p. 187). Again, there is quite a remarkable departure already from Lacan's view that even before birth we are already immersed in the Symbolic, even though the subject emerges from a mythic pre-subject represented by the delta at the bottom of the Graph of Desire. Deleuze criticised Klein's assumption of the two different positions of the unconscious (paranoid-schizoid and depressive positions), "for the very theme of positions implies the idea of the orientations of psychic life and of cardinal points; it also implies the idea of the organization of this life in accordance with variable or shifting coordinates and dimensions, an entire geography and geometry of living dimensions" (Deleuze, 1990, p. 188). The 'abyss' of the 'bottomless depth' of oral and anal drives does not enter an equilibrium via introjection and projection of 'good objects' as Klein suggested; rather, what Deleuze reads as being what the schizoid position opposes is "an organism without parts, a body without organs, with neither mouth nor anus, having given up all introjection or projection, and being complete, at this price" (Deleuze, 1990, p. 188). The 'abyss' of bodily depth enters into a relation facing a 'body' that is 'complete', or of no depth, a body of surface. It is, for Deleuze, at this point in his work, at this moment when "the tension between id and ego is formed. Two depths are opposed: a hollow depth, wherein bits whirl about and explode, and full depth" (Deleuze, 1990, p. 189). The question of a superego, the tensions between ego-id and the question of depth-surfaces are aligned with Deleuze's understanding of the body and its generative sounds that will be transformed into language. This 'creative' delineation that Deleuze offers to Klein's work, inspired by Stern and his view of infants as 'full' of life potency rather than 'lacking', also establishes a curious ethics to this ontological model and his genealogy of sense. He writes: "The superego does not begin with the first introjected objects, as Melanie Klein says, but rather with this good object which holds itself aloft. Freud often insisted on the importance of this transference from depth to height, which indicates, between the id and the superego, a total change of orientation and a central reorganization of psychic life" (Deleuze, 1990, p. 189). Between id and superego, as Deleuze reads, there is a difference in mode, since "depth has an internal tension determined by dynamic categories—container-contained, empty-full, massive-meagre, etc." (Deleuze, 1990, p. 190) all the while "the tension proper to height [meaning the superego here] is verticality, difference in size, the large and the small" (Deleuze, 1990, p. 190). He seems to be talking about different intensities or qualities, one of depth and one of the surface. The superego and the conflict it inaugurates in psychic life are, therefore, of another quality to the conflicts of depths, of the body without organs or, in a simple sense, of the drive.

To Deleuze, there are no such things as 'good objects', rather, there is an internalised superego acting as good object which the ego identifies with. Identification is, according to this view, a mechanism of surface. The level of the depressive position would then put into a halt the flux of introjections and projections, of dynamic exchanges, and substitute for it 'identification' with both internal objects and with the "object of the heights" (Deleuze, 1990, p. 192). In this sense, the 'voice from above' is the basis of 'morality', or the 'compass' of psychic life that is taken in, as it enters into a surface-depth relation towards the exploding tension of the drives.

For Deleuze, when Freud speaks of erogenous 'zones' there is already an external 'mapping' onto the body, as such zones are not 'natural' to its chaotic nature, but rather, are inscribed and delineated. "The erogenous zones are cut up on the surface of the body, around orifices marked by the presence of mucous membranes. When people note that internal organs are also able to become erogenous zones, it appears that this is conditional upon the spontaneous topology of the body" (Deleuze, 1990, p. 197). What is most important in *Logic of Sense,* therefore, is Deleuze's creative alternative to the quality of affects and the drives, interweaving body and language in a more complex, more materialist matrix than in a 'classic' Freudian or Lacanian version. Guattari, in *Chaosmosis*, from 1992, will pick up on such theory of the genesis of sense and the relation of the body, the unconscious and an expanded notion of the possibilities of signification. Guattari, as a clinician, proposes a "movement towards a polyphonic and heterogenetic comprehension of subjectivity" (Guattari, 1995a, p. 6).

Žižek (2004) considers *Logic of Sense* to be Deleuze's most important piece of writing, whilst dismissing *Anti-Oedipus* in his book *Organs Without Bodies* precisely because in this piece Deleuze works at this limit of tension between materialism and idealism, abandoning the latter altogether in favour of the former in his *Capitalism and Schizophrenia* series with Guattari. Following these two moments (*Logic of Sense* and *Anti-Oedipus*), Deleuze dives into an 'abandonment of sense' and writes about the logic of 'sensation'.

The piece in which Deleuze's exposition of sensation and, thus, vibration is more clearly connected to what we are trying to touch in anxiety appears in *Francis Bacon: The Logic of Sensation*, originally published in French in 1981, after meeting Guattari. The book, as the title suggests, goes beyond the tradition of representation in art history and finds an anchor in the work of the English painter, Francis Bacon, on the exploration of sensation. Ideas about the body, the body without organs and of the 'potency' of depth rehearsed in the second part of *Logic of Sense* can be found here again, with additional emphasis. About the body and sensation (and vibration), Deleuze's poetic, difficult, yet summarised definition is the following:

> The body without organs is opposed less to organs than to that organization of organs we call an organism. It is an intense and intensive body. It is traversed by a wave that traces levels or thresholds in the body according to the variations of its amplitude. Thus the body does not have organs, but thresholds or levels. Sensation is not qualitative and qualified, but has only an intensive reality, which no longer determines with itself representative elements, but allotropic variations. *Sensation is vibration* [my emphasis]. […] It is a whole nonorganic life, for the organism is not life, it is what imprisons life. The body is completely living, and yet nonorganic. Likewise sensation, when it acquires a body through the organism, takes on an

excessive and spasmodic appearance, exceeding the bounds of organic activity. (Deleuze, 2003, p. 45)

The notion of the 'bWo' as we can see in the above quote, by this point, is affirmative and sensorial. It is contrasted with the organism, marking a 'body' that is not of the order of the Symbolic but it also has trouble fitting into the Imaginary, aligned more with resonances of the Real. If we rescue the 'vibrational moments' in Freud and Lacan's work on anxiety, namely the excessive, the libidinal, the Id-perceptions and the Real that is not anchored in the Symbolic resonate with the 'bWo'. Deleuze, in his collaboration with Guattari, will, in fact, twist the unconscious from the perspective of the Real (Sauvagnargues, 2016), delineating possibilities for subjectivity and political life accordingly. The shared plane in which the unconscious is open to an immanent and ethical positioning along others is named an 'assemblage', a mode of togetherness in which "objects constitute themselves in a transversal, vibratory position, conferring on them a soul, a becoming ancestral, animal, vegetal, cosmic" (Guattari, 1995a, p. 102). Their ontological and ethical proposition, therefore, accounts for the possibilities of the unconscious beyond not only an individualist or family-centred model, but also beyond a human-exceptionalism framework. Vibration assumes the function of an ethical and political utopia in Guattari's 'To Have done with the Massacre of the Body', from 1973: "We want to open our bodies to the bodies of other people, to other people in general. We want to let vibrations pass among us, let energies circulate, allow desires to merge" (Guattari, 2009, p. 212).

## Deleuze and Guattari: Vibrating Together

Rather than focusing on the 'castrations' Oedipal models perceive as structural in the unconscious, Deleuze and Guattari, working together in the difficult and experimental *Capitalism and Schizophrenia* titles, published between 1972 and 1980, see the unconscious as a space of positive desire production, a space for expansion rather than a place for lack and neurotic limitations. Instead of the Mirror Stage and the realms of the Symbolic and the Imaginary—which give rise to a desire anchored in the

Other and aiming at recognition, as proposed by Lacan—they see the unconscious as 'rhizomatic' and desire as a creative force. Rejecting the 'arborescent' structure defended by psychoanalysis (a vertical, centralised, one-way model) they put forward the opposite to it: the rhizome, which undermined the very notion of structure, proposing an unconscious which is not fixed, instead multiple and fluid (Deleuze & Guattari, 1987). The rhizome is defined in a passage at the beginning of *A Thousand Plateaus*, which reads: "unlike trees or their roots, the rhizome connects any point to any other point, and its traits are not necessarily linked to traits of the same nature; it brings into play very different regimes of signs, and even nonsign states" (Deleuze & Guattari, 1987, p. 21). Rhizomes are also 'acentered', not coming from one specific point neither going to any single direction. This multiple nature allows rhizomes to ceaselessly establish "connections between semiotic chains, organisations of power, and circumstances relative to the arts, sciences, and social struggles" (Deleuze & Guattari, 1987, p. 7), an idea that seems to expand the Lacanian premises of the Imaginary and the Symbolic as having to work with their delineating limitations, granting one another the capacity to fulfil itself. Rhizomatic subjects engage with all the potentiality that 'vibrates' around them (also in them, through them, and so on), in a way "that is totally different from the arborescent relation: all manner of 'becomings'" (Deleuze & Guattari, 1987, p. 21). Desire, emerging from 'desiring-machines' through desire-production, "is at work everywhere, functioning smoothly at times, at other times in fits and starts" (Deleuze & Guattari, 1983, p. 1). For them, the meeting of desiring-machines (which derive from a non-distinctive classification between humans, nature, etc.) allows for a 'coupling' from which the interruption of one flow of desire generates another flow, in another direction, forming a rhizomatic cartography which is, inherently, multi-directional (Deleuze & Guattari, 1983). When flows of desire are interrupted, a Body without Organs emerges, presenting its "smooth, slippery, opaque, taut surface as a barrier" (Deleuze & Guattari, 1983, p. 8), subverting any notion of bodies being 'hermetically' organised. The BwO is an all-encompassing version of the organism, comprising the 'virtual' affective potentialities that a body carries with it—in a sense similar to what Lacan suggests with the Real towards the late phase of his writings (as a register which is 'unbound')—only by the engagement with this 'machine' of desire-production. A 'becoming', as described in *Anti-Oedipus*, happens when this realm of virtual potentiality is activated, in the meeting of "the process of production of the desiring-machines and the nonproductive stasis of the body without organs" (Deleuze & Guattari, 1983, p. 8). Without veering away from this archival tracing of 'vibration', it is worth mentioning that such proposition of becoming in relation to the BwO takes us back to Lygia Clark's vibrational body and its openness to *co-poiesis* in her practice.

Both in *Anti-Oedipus* and in *A Thousand Plateaus*, 'vibration' appears as part of Deleuze and Guattari's lexicon, often-times relating to their writings on art, music and literature and their potency in engendering new worlds and new aesthetic paradigms. In a passage of *Anti-Oedipus* where they critically engage with the Freudian understanding of love, sexuality and libido, vibration operates as a non-situated, collective and connecting quality of libido. To hold onto this, I will fragment this specific passage in more detail. They start by positioning psychoanalysis within a specific modern tradition that is particularly conservative, claiming, with humour, that "psychoanalysis has not made its pictorial revolution" (Deleuze & Guattari, 1983, p. 352), thus, is still attached to an 'old' aesthetic reference. The Freudian framework of Oedipus therefore modulates libido and the body within a specific political economy:

> There is a hypothesis dear to Freud: the libido does not invest the social field as such except on condition that it be desexualized and sublimated. If he holds so closely to this hypothesis, it is because he wants above all to keep sexuality in the limited framework of Narcissus and Oedipus, the ego and the family. Consequently, every sexual libidinal investment having a social dimension seems to him to testify to a pathogenic state, a "fixation" in narcissism, or a "regression" to Oedipus and to the pre-oedipal stages, by means of which homosexuality will be explained as a reinforced drive, and paranoia as a means of defense. We have seen on the contrary that what the libido invested, through its loves and sexuality, was the social field itself in its economic, political, historical, racial, and cultural determinations: in delirium the libido is continually re-creating History, continents, kingdoms, races, and cultures. Not that it is advisable to put historical representations in the place of the familial representations of the Freudian

> unconscious, or even the archetypes of a collective unconscious. (Deleuze & Guattari, 1983, p. 352)

Collectivising this modulation by extending its symbolic "essentialism", in a Jungian manner, alternatively, is not the solution either, as they hint above. Rather, they argue, libido is a matter of encounters with others, indexing social relations that cannot be reduced to 'history' (or a transcendental connecting illusion), but harnessed into a 'geohistory' (or a cartography of relations). Opening libido to the level of vibration would thus do away with the necessity of a subjectivity that is modulated within the political economy of the modern and Oedipal family, organised by its binary and phallic sexual difference. For them, "our choices in matters of love are at the crossroads of 'vibrations', which is to say that they express connections, disjunctions, and conjunctions of flows that cross through a society, entering and leaving it, linking it up with other societies, ancient or contemporary, remote or vanished, dead or yet to be born" (Deleuze & Guattari, 1983, p. 353). Libido, through the perspective of a vibrational body, thus, has an affective character and it is harnessed in the socius in a way of encounters that extend beyond the limits of a historical (and Symbolic) delineation of reality. In *Anti-Oedipus*, therefore, we can find the path contrary to the modulation of desire; or a rescuing of the early-Freud libido as harnessed to the collective rather than the socius. They write:

> But flows and codes of socius that do not portray anything, that merely *designate* zones of libidinal intensity on the body without organs, and that are emitted, captured, intercepted by the being that we are then determined to love, like a point-sign, a singular point in the entire network of the intensive body that responds to History, that vibrates with it. (Deleuze & Guattari, 1983, p. 353)

In *A Thousand Plateaus*, vibration appears as synonymous to 'becomings' in the 'plane of consistency'. We can move beyond the early-Freud libidinal excess theory into finding here resonances to what Lacan hints without theorising in his later conceptualisation of the Real. Instead of operating in a logic of 'two' (as the planes made possible by, for example, the modulating libidinal economy of psychoanalysis), multiplicities are kept alive in what they call a 'plane of consistency', defining that:

> Far from reducing the multiplicities' number of dimensions to two, the plane of consistency cuts across them all, intersects them in order to bring into coexistence any number of multiplicities, with any number of dimensions. The plane of consistency is the intersection of all concrete forms. Therefore all becomings are written like sorcerers' drawings on this plane of consistency, which is the ultimate Door providing a way out for them. This is the only criterion to prevent them from bogging down, or veering into the void. (Deleuze & Guattari, 1987, p. 251)

It is at this level, of the plane of consistency, that the 'imperceptible' can be 'seen and heard', that vibrations are located. Vibration, therefore, is a quality of affect. If we return to earlier pages and to Deleuze's course on Spinoza and affect, the collective and non-representational aspects of affect are again rescued in 'vibration'. Vibration, accordingly, resonates affectively, opening up to what is not known, which is not divided in two, keeping multiplicity alive. It is also "where the imperceptible is seen and heard", when the body is open to sensation, even the most subtle ones.

Interestingly, the body in its materiality and capacity for sensation versus a cognitive self-consciousness will again be linked with vibration in their last co-authored book—risking slight dualistic undertones, they still extrapolate the complex entanglement between concept and matter, echoing Deleuze's reading of Spinoza's theory of affects as still relational, as mentioned. The final account of the pair Deleuze and Guattari on vibration appears in *What is Philosophy?,* first published in 1991. In this piece, again, vibration is utilised in relation to music, philosophy and art, but there is one specific passage that connects vibration with the materiality of the 'I', the brain and nervous system and the field of the 'other'. They write:

> It is the brain that says *I,* but *I* is an other. It is not the same brain as the brain of connections and secondary integrations, although there is no transcendence here. And this *I* is not only the "I conceive" of the brain as philosophy, it is also the "I feel" of the brain as art. Sensation is no less brain

> than the concept. If we consider the nervous connections of excitation-reaction and the integrations of perception action, we need not ask at what stage on the path or at what level sensation appears, for it is presupposed and withdrawn. The withdrawal is not the opposite but a correlate of the survey. Sensation is excitation itself, not insofar as it is gradually prolonged and passes into the reaction but insofar as it is preserved or preserves its vibrations. (Deleuze & Guattari, 1994, p. 211)

It is clear that the I, or the subject of consciousness and enunciation, speaks to that level of subjectivity which is not only conscious but which is actualised through language. What I find particular compelling about their addition to vibration and sensation here is how it echoes yet again what Freud hinted at in his 'An Outline of Psychoanalysis', from 1938, namely the quality of the Id as being capable of perceptions that extend beyond the ego and consciousness. Here, then, it becomes clear how vibration is an unconscious sensation.

For Deleuze and Guattari, as this genealogy of the notion of vibration makes very clear, subjectivity extends to the level of 'sensation', or the level of 'vibration'. Their final definition of vibration addresses precisely this almost 'materiality' of the unconscious; or, as contemporary Lacanians would express it, how the unconscious is the speaking-body:

> Sensation contracts the vibrations of the stimulant on a nervous surface or in a cerebral volume: what comes before has not yet disappeared when what follows appears. This is its way or responding to chaos. Sensation itself vibrates because it contracts vibrations. It preserves itself because it preserves vibrations: it is Monument. It resonates because it makes its harmonics resonate. Sensation is the contracted vibration that has become quality, variety. That is why the brain-subject is here called *soul* or *force,* since only the soul preserves by contracting that which matter dissipates, or radiates, furthers, reflects, refracts, or converts. (Deleuze & Guattari, 1994, p. 211)

In their complex cosmologic assemblage, vibrations of the world are constant, captured by 'sensation', which is a capacity of the I that goes beyond 'knowledge' and beyond 'feeling'. If we add a Lacanian layer to this, we can place 'sensation' at the level of an affective Real, rather than the Symbolic (knowledge) or the Imaginary (feelings).

## Vibrating the Clinic

Guattari's solo meditations and theoretical production were as ambitious and consistent as those he imparted with Deleuze in *Capitalism and Schizophrenia*. His writings reflect the onto-epistemic twists proposed by Deleuze, and focus on what he calls 'schizoanalytic cartographies' and a 'diagrammatic' mode of thought. The kernel of his contributions relates to the possibilities of a 'vibrational' Real.

The Real in Guattari is not confined to the margins of representation, as a negative of the 'phenomenological' Thing, as a structuralist-minded understanding of early to mid-life Lacan insists on, and late-Lacan perhaps leaves open ended (Guattari, 1995b). Guattari worked on a detailed transdisciplinary project of semiotics, metamodeling and expression in his solo writing before, during and after his encounter with Deleuze. He sought inspiration in the linguistic theory of 'Glossematics', from the Danish linguist Hjelmslev and his semiotic matrix of polyvocality, which, differently to the Saussurean model of linguistics that inspired Lacan, offers scope for the expression of a-signifying ruptures, rather than confining them as a negative to the 'bivocality' of representation. To Guattari, "the subjectivity produced in the world of signification is a shut-in, a semiological shipwreck" (Genosko, 2002, p. 168), in which "polyvocity becomes bi[uni]vocity" (Genosko, 2002, p. 169). In his published personal notebooks *The Anti-Oedipus Papers* (2006) and in *A Thousand Plateaus*, co-authored with Deleuze, several references to the question of expression beyond the possibilities of representation are made. Guattari's model of the subject also expands Hjelmslev's linguistic ideas to 'matter'/'substance', including not only the social and the political as well as the ecological and the biological into a common matrix of affectability, or into a metamodeling of the 'machine'. Janell Watson, a scholar of Guattari's complex diagrammatic thinking, writes that "the political potential of Guattari's semiotic matrix lies in its refusal to let go of the real, as does Lacan by focusing on a signifier which cannot possibly even 'represent' the real. Guattari's matrix can include the real because it does not confine itself to the domain of representation—in other words, the small ellipsis of language" (Watson, 2008, para.44). Such 'diagrammatic' thought, moving beyond the possibilities of representation and non-representation, shakes completely the Lacanian primacy of the Symbolic for subjective formation, which is implied in Lacanian topological models (until the 1970s, at least). As such, "forging a path of access to the real opens up political possibilities, whereas blocking out the real shuts down politics. The capitalist and psychoanalytic politics of signification which upholds the tyranny of the signifier in turn preserves the domination of the ruling classes" (Watson, 2008, para.44). This dense theoretical twist has powerful clinical implications—it opens space for a 'nomadic ethics' (Braidotti, 2006a), or for 'becomings' rather than 'beings' in the psychoanalytic clinic.

The clinical model practiced by Guattari on the back of his collaboration with Deleuze and his connection with the Institutional Psychotherapy movement in France (known as schizoanalysis) is thus a practice of 'becomings' (Robcis, 2021). For them, when dealing with the unconscious, "it is not the lines of pressure that matter, but on the contrary the lines of escape" (Deleuze & Guattari, 1983, p. 338), lines of flight, of movement. Instead of a clinic focused on the power of repression (and foreclosure and disavowal, as the psychotic and perverse core mechanisms in the Lacanian clinic), schizoanalysis works with the power of the 'lines of flight'. For them "the unconscious does not apply pressure to consciousness; rather, consciousness applies pressure and strait-jackets the unconscious, to prevent its escape" (Deleuze & Guattari, 1983, p. 338). Thus being, the lines of flight, the moments of inventiveness and creativity not only in the symptom but in the *sinthôme*, is what keeps one alive and is the key to a clinic of becoming (Biehl & Locke, 2017). As a clinical practitioner, 'thinking-with' (rather than 'against') these theorists enables me to move beyond discursivity in what concerns the 'grammar of suffering' in the case of anxiety (Dunker, 2015), thinking of the materiality of the body, and life, in light of the ontological turn in medical anthropology (Mol, 2002; Biehl, 2005). Unconscious 'lines of flight' meet a 'common' (Federici, 2019, 2020) 'nomadic affectivity' (Braidotti, 2006b).

For this reason, the influence of Deleuze and Guattari in the Brazilian Psychiatric Reform, for example, is notorious. Aside from the historical fact that Guattari visited Brazil during the period of re-democratisation after the Military Dictatorship relinquished in the early 1980s, taking part in critical psychiatric meetings, the schizoanalytic model finds, to this day resonances in the public mental health care system (Amarante & Nunes, 2018). As asylums started to be closed, following an international trend of psychiatric reform in the 1980s, outpatient 'psychosocial support centres' (CAPS) were established nationally after the year 2000. The centrality of music and art therapy, as well as the importance of community care and psychosocial work in 'territories' in Brazilian public mental health, is frequently justified 'schizoanalytically'. Arriscado Nunes and Siqueira-Silva (2016) argue that this schizoanalytic appropriation in the Brazilian Psychiatric Reform confers a decolonial quality to its practices, once suffering, ruptures and the production of meaning are bound to the community and to a local temporality, rather than enclosed within hegemonic (and colonial) psychiatric frames or psychoanalytic models. Accordingly, the clinical reverberations of schizoanalysis are also present in the ontological turn observed within medical anthropology (Mol, 2002), challenging universalising dominant health epistemologies that offer little or no space for the multiple performances and experiences of illness, suffering, health and the body.[9]

The ruptures characteristic of psychic suffering and 'madness' (psychoses, more often) need, according to the schizoanalytic model, to be supported with grounds of expression that are not enclosed to individual psychotherapy and psychiatric care (in other words, not forced into the limits of being, but open to multiple becomings). Rather, the expression of such unconscious ruptures needs to be collective and territorialised in the community, crossing aesthetic, sensorial and political zones of affect (Lancetti, 2015). That is what Guattari (2015) called a clinical model of 'transversality'. The transversal moves the centre of the axis of enunciation from the subject and their triangular relation with the Other and the

[9] The Brazilian CAPS model of community mental health care features in a very recent report on Global Mental Health issued by the World Health Organization in June 2021 that is the result of an effort to promote person-centred and rights-based approaches in the heavily over-medicalised and still violent field of mental health care (WHO, 2021). This model, albeit precarious in reality, is anchored in co-production, active participation of service users in all decision-making, the right to choose and negotiate a treatment alongside a multidisciplinary team and a strong local community support system of networks of care.

analyst, challenging the power structure (or colonising violence) sustained by the classic transferential relation in psychoanalysis. Instead of relying on the fixity of psychic structures (neurosis, psychosis and perversion)—which stems off Lacan's linguistic logic (and the representation versus non-representation binary of this linguistic model)—or on the function of interpretations that are Oedipally inscribed (with sexual difference, the family drama and castration at its core)—a plural and situated clinic is proposed. Whilst there is significant literature on the influence of Deleuze and Guattari in the Brazilian Psychiatric reform in relation to psychosis (similarly to the legacy of French Institutional Psychotherapy, see Robcis, 2021), little is offered in relation to the potential of the schizoanalytic model in the clinic of anxiety. What the archival mobilisation allows us to do is to extend the clinical value of unconscious 'lines of flight' into the clinic of anxiety.

In Guattari's practice, the commitment to the 'lines of flight' is apparent in the institutional mobilisation of what we can call now the 'full-void' into *co-poiesis.* Guattari (1998) has offered a rich account of how such power relations were challenged in practice at the clinic of La Borde in his essay '*La Grille*'. The 'grid' of activities and function was fundamental to the emergency of 'deregulation frames' *(cadrer le dérèglements)* that would act as a system of articulation of all the patients, staff and space, allowing for the "invention of a [new] language". The set of relations and their non-hierarchical arrangements of the clinic were fundamental to the treatment to mostly cases of psychoses at La Borde. In defending this model of clinical practice psychosocially, the question to be worked out is not just of the macropolitical effects of the 'pimping of life' (Rolnik, 2019), but of its 'molecular' dynamics, as Guattari (2000) argues in *The Three Ecologies.* Following Denise Ferreira da Silva (2016), who proposes that such an ethico-political project does not entail simply tracing 'differences' and the effects of difference for what they are (a strategy of thinking she calls 'critique'), even when providing an intersectional feminist critique; rather, it is matter of moving beyond 'separating' estrangements and proposing 'entanglements' instead.[10] In other words, clinically engaging at the molecular level means not only speaking of the 'effects' of the logic of the Same/One across human multiplicities; nor does it involve thinking radically through a psychoanalytic archive whilst still succumbing the Real, ruptures, a-signification and affects, such as anxiety, to the limits of universalist signifiers and a corresponding Symbolic structure.

As such, going back to Guattari's polyvocal Real, we can trace what I am gathering as Guattari's 'theory of anxiety'. The ruptures of a vibrational Real add a particular nuance to Guattari's understanding of anxiety, a conceptualisation he does not develop in detail but that he insinuates in various moments. Guattari places 'anguish' within the domain of the ruptures—beyond the limits of bivocality—which, in his critique of psychoanalysis and 'Integrated World Capitalism'—his own vocabulary for neoliberal capitalism—is prevented from operating its 'surprise'. He writes:

> Everything that pertains to the domain of rupture, surprise, and anguish, but also desire, the will to love and to create, somehow has to fit into the registers of dominant references. There is always an arrangement ready to prevent anything that might be of a dissident nature in thought and desire. There is an attempt to eliminate what I call the processes of singularization. Everything that surprises, however mildly, has to be classifiable in some area of framing or reference. (Guattari & Rolnik, 2007, pp. 58–59)

The psychoanalytic (and, we can add, the psychodiagnosis that extended through the twentieth century) *modus operadi* is, to Guattari, one of such frames that modulates anguish and its ruptures under the Modern shadow of subjectivity. Affects and anguish are contextually modulated and our relation to them is indicative of our cartographical

[10] Denise Ferreira da Silva writes: "Why not assume that beyond their physical (bodily and geographic) conditions of existence, in their fundamental constitutions, at the subatomic level, humans exist entangled with everything else (animate and in-animate) in the universe). Why not conceive of human differences—the ones nineteenth and twentieth century anthropologists and sociologists selected as fundamental human descriptors—as effects of both spacetime conditions and a knowledge program modelled after Newtonian (nineteenth century anthropology) and Einsteinian (twentieth century social scientific knowledge) physics, in which separability is the privileged ontological principal. Without separability, difference among human groups and between human and nonhuman entities, has a very limited explanatory purchase and ethical significance" (Ferreira da Silva, 2016, pp. 64–65).

positioning, Guattari writes: "every individual and social group conveys its own system of modelising subjectivity; that is, a certain cartography—composed of cognitive references as well as mythical, ritual and symptomatological references—with which it positions itself in relation to its affects and anguishes, and attempts to manage its inhibitions and drives" (Guattari, 1995a, p. 11). Anguish, or anxiety, by being situated within the domain of a-signifying ruptures are not reduceable to the binary (representability versus non-representability) logic of the Symbolic as anchored over the paradigm of 'lack'.

Guattari makes this argument clearer in a note entitled 'Of Anxiety, the Phallic Object and Interpretation', published as part of his *Anti-Oedipus Papers.* There Guattari places anxiety as "the intermixture of two intersecting drives—Faithfulness to polyvocal remainders (the mother) (adhesion to the remainders, adherence to the Lacanian 'a')—Desire for bi-univocal oedipal normality" (Guattari, 2006, p. 103). In a diagram I am nicknaming 'Guattari's Graph of Anxiety', Guattari maps 'eros' (or affect, jouissance, libido, for him) as extending beyond the death-drive that anchors attachment to bi-univocality. He proposes a small circle of 'bi-univocality' is anchored by the death drive; a larger circle wraps it in its middle, this larger one anchored by polyvocality and headed by eros. The unconscious (Eros) is thus moored by polyvocality—or multiple possibilities of enunciation, expression or representation that do not fit into any Symbolic structure or arrangement. What this implies is that the affect of anxiety is not reducible to interpretation, nor indexed to a relation to the Phallic Law-of-the-Father, Oedipus and the Other that anchor the Symbolic. What this diagram, followed by this study on vibration, enables us to map is that Guattari offers a complementing theory of anxiety that Freud and Lacan only hinted at but were not able to clearly delineate. What we see here is the potency of anxiety in a clinic that encounters the subject anxious, at the edge of their being, but not yet open to novel becomings.

Following the trail of 'vibration' through the oeuvre of Deleuze and Guattari, affect is an ethical disposition that is collectively produced. Affect vibrates beyond the confines of an individual and the Symbolic frame that modulates one's experience of such affects. We have arrived at this ethical framing of the subject in Deleuze and Guattari by pursuing a cartographic genealogy of the concept of vibration, discussing how it is crucial to the understanding of notions of 'sensation' and of 'affect' within this tradition of thinking. Anxiety, as an affect of rupture, exceeds the modulation of the bivocality of possibilities assumed by the psychoanalytic model and, as such, is inscribed in the plane of the 'commons', following Federici (2019, 2020); or of a nomadic ethics (Braidotti, 2006a) instead of a logic of 'difference with separability' and domination (Ferreira da Silva, 2016). In other words, possibilities for 'becomings' rather than 'beings' in the psychoanalytic clinic.

Returning to the critique presented earlier in the book—which point at a process of 'dividualisation' (Deleuze, 1992) in the process of diagnosis and treatment of anxiety, extending such alienation to a psychoanalytic orientation that is restricted to the possibilities of 'being', rather than of 'becoming'—what proves necessary is an encounter between the common, the affective, collective, ethical disposition rescued in the concept of 'vibration', and psychoanalytic possibilities. How can we conceive an understanding of anxiety in psychoanalysis that is not dividualising? Can psychoanalysis work with an unconscious that vibrates? This is what I move into arguing, shifting from anxiety and its estrangement, as we have set out in the beginning, to a possible entanglement, as we will conclude.

## References


Ahmed, S. (2004). *The Cultural Politics of Emotion*. Routledge.

Alaimo, S. (2014). Thinking as the Stuff of the World. *O-ZONE: A journal of Object-Oriented Studies., 1*, 13–21.

Amarante, P., & Nunes, M. O. (2018). A reforma psiquiátrica no SUS e a luta por uma sociedade sem manicômios. *Ciência & Saúde Coletiva, 23*(6), 2067–2074.

Arriscado Nunes, J., & Siqueira-Silva, R. (2016). Dos "abismos do inconsciente" as razões da diferença: criação estética e descolonização da desrazão na Reforma Psiquiátrica Brasileira. *Sociologias*. Ano 18, *43* (September/December), 208–237

Biehl, J. (2005). *Vita: Life in a Zone of Social Abandonment*. University of California Press.

Biehl, J., & Locke, P. (2017). *Unfinished: The Anthropology of Becoming*. Duke University Press.

Braidotti, R. (1994). *Nomadic Subjects: Embodiment and Sexual Difference in Contemporary Feminist Theory*. Columbia University Press.

Braidotti, R. (2006a). *Transpositions: On Nomadic Ethics*. Polity Press.

Braidotti, R. (2006b). Affirming the Affirmative: On Nomadic Affectivity. *Rhizome*. Issue 11/12 (Fall 2005/Spring2006). [Online]. http://www.rhizomes.net/issue11/braidotti.html

Braidotti, R. (2011). *Nomadic Theory. The Portable Rosi Braidotti*. Columbia University Press.

Braidotti, R. (2013, June 19). Conversation with Rosi Braidotti. *nY.* [Online]. https://www.ny-web.be/artikels/conversation-rosi-braidotti/

Braidotti, R. (2017). *Per Una Politica Affermativa*. Mimesis Edizioni.

Braidotti, R. (2019). *Posthuman Knowlegde*. Polity.

Brousse, M. H. (2007). Hysteria and Sinthôme. In V. Voruz & B. Wolf (Eds.), *The Late Lacan, An Introduction*. State University of New York Press.

David-Menard, M. (2014). *Deleuze e a psicanálise*. Civilização Brasileira.

Deleuze, G. (1968). *Spinoza et le problème de l'expression*. Les Éditions de Minuit.

Deleuze, G. (1978). Sur Spinoza Cours Vincennes—St Denis, Cours du January 24. [Online]. https://www.webdeleuze.com/cours/spinoza

Deleuze, G. (1981). *Spinoza—Philosophie pratique*. Les Éditions de Minuit.

Deleuze, G. (1990). *Logic of Sense*. The Athlone Press.

Deleuze, G. (1991). *Bergsonism*. Zone Books.

Deleuze, G. (1992). Postscript on Societies of Control. *October, 59*, 3–7.

Deleuze, G. (1995). *Difference and Repetition*. Columbia University Press.

Deleuze, G. (2003). *Francis Bacon: The Logic of Sensation*. University of Minnesota Press.

Deleuze, G., & Guattari, F. (1983). *Anti-Oedipus—Capitalism and Schizophrenia*. University of Minnesota Press.

Deleuze, G., & Guattari, F. (1987). *A Thousand Plateaus—Capitalism and Schizophrenia*. University of Minnesota Press.

Deleuze, G., & Guattari, F. (1994). *What is Philosophy?* Columbia University Press.

Deleuze, G., & Parnet, C. (1987). *Dialogues*. Columbia University Press.

Dosse, F. (2010). *Gilles Deleuze & Félix Guattari: Intersecting Lives*. Columbia University Press.

Dunker, C. (2015). *Mal-Estar, Sofrimento e Sintoma*. Boitempo Editorial.

Federici, S. (2019). *Re-enchanting the World: Feminism and the Politics of the Commons*. PM Press/Kairos.

Federici, S. (2020). *Beyond the Periphery of the Skin: Rethinking, Remaking, and Reclaiming the Body in Contemporary Capitalism*. PM Press/Kairos.

Felman, S. (1982). *Literature and Psychoanalysis: The Question of Reading: Otherwise*. Johns Hopkins University Press.

Ferreira da Silva, D. (2016). On Difference Without Separability. Catalogue of the 32nd *São Paulo Art Biennial 'Incerteza Viva'*, 57–65.

Genosko, G. (2002). *Félix Guattari: An aberrant Introduction*. Continuum.

Gil, J. (1998). *Metamorphoses of the Body*. University of Minnesota Press.

Grosz, E. (2007). Deleuze, Bergson and the Concept of Life. *Revue internationale de philosophie, 241*(3), 287–300.

Guattari, F. (1995a). *Chaosmosis. An Ethico-aesthetic paradigm*. Indiana University Press.

Guattari, F. (1995b). *The Machinic Unconscious: Essays in Schizoanalysis*. Semiotext (e).

Guattari, F. (1998). La "grille". *Chimères. Revue des schizoanalyses, 34*(Automne), 7–20.

Guattari, F. (2000). *The Three Ecologies*. The Athlone Press.

Guattari, F. (2006). *Anti-Oedipus Papers*. Semiotext(e).

Guattari, F. (2009). *Chaosophy: Texts and Interviews 1972–1977*. Semiotext(e).

Guattari, F. (2015). *Psychoanalysis and Transversality: Texts and Interviews 1955–1971*. Semiotext (e).

Guattari, F., & Rolnik, S. (2007). *Molecular Revolution in Brazil*. Semiotext(e).

Hemmings, C. (2005). Invoking Affect: Cultural theory and the ontological turn. *Cultural Studies, 19*, 548–567.

Lacan, J. (1975). *Seminar XXIII*, lesson of the 18th of November, 1975. Gallagher's translation. [Online]. http://www.lacaninireland.com/web/wp-content/uploads/2010/06/THE-SEMINAR-OF-JACQUES-LACAN-XXIII.pdf

Lancetti, A. (2015). *Contrafissura e Plasticidade Psíquica*. Hucitec Editora.

Leys, R. (2017). *The Ascent of Affect: Genealogy and Critique*. University of Chicago Press.

Malabou, C. (2016). Before and Above: Spinoza and Symbolic Necessity. *Critical Inquiry, 43*(1), 84–109.

Martin, E. (2013). 'The Potentiality of Ethnography and the Limits of Affect Theory. *Current Anthropology, 54*, 149 158.

Massumi, B. (2015). *The Politics of Affect*. Polity.

Miller, J. A. (2014). The Unconscious and the Speaking Body. *World Association of Psychoanalysis.* [Online]. https://wapol.org/en/articulos/Template.asp?intTipoPagina=4&intPublicacion=13&intEdicion=9&intIdiomaPublicacion=2&intArticulo=2742&intIdiomaArticulo=2
Moder, G. (2017). *Hegel and Spinoza: Substance and Negativity.* Northwestern University Press.
Mol, A. (2002). *The Body Multiple: Ontology in Medical Practice.* Duke University Press.
Preciado, P. B. (2018). La isquierda bajo la piel. Um prólogo para Suely Rolnik. In S. Rolnik (Ed.), *Esferas da Insurreição: notas para uma vida não cafetinada.* n-1.
Preciado, P. B. (2020). *Je suis um Monstre qui vous parle. Rapport pour une academie de psychanalystes.* Bernard Grasset.
Robcis, C. (2021). *Disalienation: Politics, Philosophy, and Radical Psychiatry in Postwar France.* University of Chicago Press.
Rolnik, S. (2019). *Esferas da Insurreição: notas para uma vida não cafetinada.* n-1.
Sauvagnargues, A. (2016). *Artmachines: Deleuze, Guattari, Simondon.* Edinburgh University Press.
Schuster, A. (2016). *The Trouble with Pleasure. Deleuze and Psychoanalysis.* The MIT Press.
Tomkins, S. S., & Smith, B. (1995). *Exploring Affect: The Selected Writings of Silvan S Tomkins.* Cambridge University Press.
Wahl, J. (2016). *Human Existence and Transcendence.* University of Notre Dame Press.
Watson, J. (2008). Schizoanalysis as Metamodeling. *Fibreculture* (12). [Online]. https://twelve.fibreculturejournal.org/fcj-077-schizoanalysis-as-metamodeling/
WHO. (2021). Guidance on Community Mental Health Services: Promoting person-centred and Rights-based Approaches. *World Health Organization,* June. [Online]. https://www.who.int/publications/i/item/guidance-and-technical-packages-on-community-mental-health-services
Žižek, S. (2004). *Organs Without Bodies: On Deleuze and Consequences.* Routledge.
Žižek, S. (2010). *Interrogating the Real.* Continuum.
Žižek, S. (2017). *Incontinence of the Void: Economico-Philosophical Spandrels.* Short Circuit.

# 9

# Conclusion: Co-Poiesis on the Couch

In order to approach the question '*What can anxiety do?*', we have explored the possibilities and impossibilities of this encounter with the Real, this excessive affect, in psychoanalytic praxis. And we have done so by naming this encounter a vibration. Anxiety, according to this hypothesis, vibrates through me that which extends beyond me or my grasp. In this book, we arrive at vibration via the work of Lygia Clark and her critique of the 'limits of the Plane' and the possibilities of a frontier 'full-void', as her understanding of the common bodily unconscious in her 'Structuring of the Self' (1976–1988) series.

Vibration is the conceptual artifice we utilise in order to be able to think of affects beyond the individual, beyond the Oedipal frame, beyond Symbolic-Imaginary realms, beyond ego-to-ego relations and a short-circuit of bodily jouissance. As such, Clark's 'full-void' reorients the Real. Vibration, as we learn with Suely Rolnik (2000), is the ethical capacity of affect recombination, creativity and a model of political ontology that is in tune with contemporary epistemological, ecological and political demands—namely, an interdependent, entangled horizon of subjectivity and bio-politics. Vibration is a term I mobilise not only from the artistic practice of Lygia Clark, but also in its roots in Deleuze and Guattari's rich


A. C. Minozzo, *Anxiety as Vibration*, Studies in the Psychosocial,
https://doi.org/10.1007/978-3-031-62856-6_9

commentaries on psychoanalysis, which I am bringing to a discussion on the contemporary status of anxiety.

Anxiety as vibration is an understanding of anxiety as not just a matter of a 'transindividual' subjectivity (which necessarily depends on recognition vis-à-vis the Other), rather, it allows me to conceptualise an entangled, affected subject. By doing so, I offer a psycho-political frame for the clinic that moves beyond the affective alienation of 'being', seeking in the rupture of anxiety not only a ground for a dialectic recognition, rather, working with the rupture of anxiety as compost for a 'common' ground. As a theoretical contribution, it is a move that enables me to work within psychoanalytic praxis whilst going beyond the level of 'critique' and embarking on the possibilities of 'creativity'. As Braidotti puts it, in an interview: "Critique ties you to the present (diagnosis, resistance, cartographies) but creativity is the future. Creativity projects you into where we're going next. Critique and creativity imply different temporal frameworks" (Braidotti, 2013). My psychosocial thinking is situated thus within this double vision of both critique and creativity, a tension I hold on to throughout this cartographic effort. In this sense, Tosquelles' militant political 'prophecy' entails a creative gaining of unconsciousness.

By theorising anxiety as an entangled vibration, this affect assumes a possibility of opening a way into a 'gaining of unconsciousness' (Tosquelles, 1991), acting, in this psychosocial cartography, as the threshold between subjective, theoretical and clinical critique and creativity. In sum, I mobilise anxiety as the looking-glass, in order to think through a psychoanalytic praxis beyond the 'pimping of Life' (Rolnik, 2017). Anxiety is the affect I work with in the search for a critique of the dividualising residues in psychoanalysis of the Freudian and Lacanian orientations, moving towards a possible creative clinic, inspired by Guattari and Lygia Clark, where rupture is co-assembled, rather than in-dividualised within the psycho-politics of alienation grounded in the orbit of the Oedipal Other. Creativity opens the affect of anxiety, in its clinical and conceptual manifestations, into the germination of new modes of living, into *sinthômes*.

In other words, this cartography follows the complex path of a formulation of anxiety as a vibration, taking it from estrangement to entanglement. The conclusion lays on a practice that works not with interpretation but with *co-poiesis*—a poetic, collective, generative construction that departs from affect, resisting domination and moving towards situated ways of existing.

## Negativity and Affirmation: Staying with this Trouble

Lacan's elaboration of the subject through (post-)structuralist lenses has made clear a certain 'politicisation' of the psychoanalytic subject, smashing, in the words of Rosi Braidotti, "any illusion of atomized individuality by embedding the subject in the thick materiality of a symbolic system of which language is the most available source. [Allowing] for subtler analyses of the interaction between self and society and among different selves than liberal, ego-based psychology" (Braidotti, 2006a, p. 18). Yet, an integral part of the model of subjectivity proposed by Lacan comes with 'negativity', or a 'lack' as its anchor. The debate around the centrality of lack in psychoanalysis is not new in feminist theory (see Brennan, 1989); whilst a clear contrast with an 'affirmative' model of the subject takes shape through the theoretical influence of Deleuze and Guattari to the fields of psychoanalysis, philosophy, the arts and humanities in more general terms.

Both 'negativity' and 'affirmation'—or 'immanence' of desire—may carry radical politics within themselves as conceptual frames through which we can think subjectivity, the psyche and, as is my concern here, the status and potencies of anxiety. Such radical potential should not be brushed off in search of a 'neat' philosophy of psychoanalysis (even if then remaining very faithful to Freudian or Lacanian teachings); that is an approach to knowledge Lacan famously rebuked in his Seminar XVII *The Other Side of Psychoanalysis* (delivered between 1969–1970), one that he called the discourse of the 'master'. In this book, my aim has been not to stretch a detailed argument for or against negativity, for or against affirmation of desire as many scholars have done (from David-Menard, 2014 to Schuster, 2016 or Nedoh & Zevnik, 2017). That would be a theoretical exercise of value, especially to philosophy, but one which can turn easily ideological and sour—a way of approaching psychoanalysis that according to Guattari, in *The Three Ecologies*, from 1989, "tends to the ornamental garden of psychoanalysis". Rather, I remain faithful to psychoanalysis' radical potential, which to me means the impossibility of 'total' knowledge of either oneself or the other; which can be translated as an ethics of the encounter that is not reliant on 'intersubjectivity' in the object relational sense but on the challenges of relations among divided subjects and how this plays out in the clinical setting. Following Frosh (2006), I hold on to the value of the 'critique' of totalising models present in Freudian and Lacanian psychoanalysis, once "what is preserved in the Lacanian critique of the object relational tendency of most contemporary psychoanalysis is one of the more radical elements of psychoanalytic thought: a pessimism concerning the possibility of positive knowledge as against negative knowledge, or critique" (Frosh, 2006, p. 20). Being truthful to this spirit means to constantly rethink psychoanalytic ideas, theories and practice in light of an always changing—and plural, multiple—world (or worlds). This is an effort Braidotti (2013) has called 'creativity'; or the production of new systems of reference, opening to the creation of new repertoires of worlds, rather than an attachment to (a stunningly male and white) dialectics of desire as lack in the heart of subjectivity and the notion of 'critique'.

In the clinic we encounter vibrant examples of negativity: from symptoms that repeat, unhealed losses that act as magnets of pain, traumatic excesses that drain and spin like a washing machine to the nonexistence of a 'sexual rapport', imaginary fantasies, a satisfaction that never comes and enigmas of the body that challenge the medical dictionaries but still, for all the suffering these generate, are able to sustain life in some way, resisting domination. A domination such that can stem both from the power of a disciplinary society, as described by Foucault (2008a, 2008b); and from a discreet and pervasive society of control, as elaborated by Deleuze (1992) as well as embodied external perpetrators, internalised super-egoic punishments or even collective disasters. Yet, even at the heart of 'negativity' there is something 'positive' that keeps going—or some 'difference' in 'repetition', as Deleuze (1995) would argue in the late 1960s.

Following Lacan's very early teachings, specially Seminars I and II, and his 'beef' with ego-analysts and post-Freudians at the time, we can be convinced to accept the non-adaptability of the subject, which relies on a singular Real that cannot be reduced to any Imaginary delineation nor any Symbolic frame (Ruti, 2012). Identification with the analyst and a strengthening of one's ego defences towards better 'adaptability' to reality was, to Lacan, in these early seminars, an ideological misinterpretation of the Freudian revolution. Insisting, therefore, in the non-adaptability of the subject (Van Haute, 2002), Lacan proposes the divided subject anchored on a 'negativity' of desire. This model of 'negativity' in Lacanian teachings, especially in the very early ones, as reflected in texts published as part of his *Écrits,* is heavily influenced by Kojéve's course on Hegel, which relies on the negativity of Desire as a guarantor of 'Self-Consciousness' or an I/Being. Kojéve starts his course on Hegel's 1807 *Phenomenology of the Spirit* with the contentious affirmation:

> Man is Self-Consciousness. He is conscious of himself, conscious of his human reality and dignity; and it is in this that he is essentially different from animals, which do not go beyond the level of simple Sentiment of self. Man becomes conscious of himself at the moment when—for the "first" time—he says "I". To understand man by understanding his "origin", is, therefore, to understand the origin of the I revealed in speech. (Kojéve, 1969, p. 3)

This 'Man' revealed in speech as 'self-consciousness' comes through a negativity in desire, for Kojéve and Hegel. Lacan takes this model onboard in his Seminar V *Formations of the Unconscious*, delivered between 1957 and 1958, where a dialectics of desire gives consistency to subjectivity beyond 'consciousness'. In Lacan, the ego will essentially be a 'misrecognition' or a mirage of the subject; a subject also crossed by discursive/social/political forces and by an excessive Real. It is in this founding 'negativity' of desire that 'action' and thus transformation of reality can happen (a formative part of Kojéve's course on Hegel taken in by Lacan). Alenka Zupančič (2012) calls this negativity that founds 'being' a 'gap' of 'with-without'. She does this by thinking through Freud's essay 'On Negation' (1925), which famously carries the possibility of a presence in absence in speech. Negativity is not then an empty hole but an airy void, or a 'gap' that makes subjectivity possible.

Thus, as discussed by Frosh (2006), in light of Rustin (1995), thinking of 'negativity' and 'positivity' (as well as affirmation, immanence and nomadism) as markers of psychoanalytic approaches and politics is one of many forms of politicising psychoanalysis. Frosh writes: "Differentiating between 'negative' and 'positive' traditions in psychoanalysis is only, of course, one possible take on the variety of ways in which the psychoanalytic field can be divided up" (Frosh, 2006, p. 21). And completes: "Nevertheless, it is a powerful one, reflecting the complexity of the critical positions taken up by psychoanalysis and the alternative possibilities of different attitudes towards therapeutic, political or cultural change" (Frosh, 2006, p. 21). In such a non-adaptability of the subject (Van Haute, 2002), which is the cornerstone of Lacanian psychoanalysis, 'negativity' and 'positivity', or rather, 'affirmation' and immanence, meet and we stay with this trouble by thinking of the Real as an 'excess', or a beyond-the-subject that is affective, entangled and collective, as proposed by Guattari (1989; Guattari & Rolnik, 2007). It is in one's excess beyond oneself that affirmation insists, according to feminist post-humanist critiques, such as that of Braidotti (2006a, 2006b, 2017), as she unpacks the modern humanist (and colonial-patriarchal) logic behind the constitution of a relation to reality, knowledge and being that German Idealism (Hegel and Kant, as her critique goes) produced and psychoanalysis still reproduces. Following this logic and when situating psychoanalysis epistemologically, historically and politically, such a 'lack' doesn't hold. Rather, negativity becomes the mark of a situated neurotic (European, male, etc.) ontological delineation (Ettinger, 2019).[1] Deleuze and Guattari's *Capitalism and Schizophrenia*, from 1972 and 1980, addresses exactly this problem, offering an explosion of psychoanalysis from within (from the triangular Oedipus to rhizomatic thousand plateaus). *Anti-Oedipus*, the first volume of the *Capitalism and Schizophrenia* series, can be considered an extension of the Lacanian endeavour, taking his

[1] Chiara Zamboni (2004) furthers the debate between transcendence and immanence as an artificial and specifically patriarchal philosophical dichotomy that feminism—and the *pratica di partire da sé,* of Italian feminism—does away with in its ethics.

critiques to mainstream psychiatry and psychoanalysis even further (Dosse, 2010).

If we consider Canguilhem's critiques of psychology, touching both on the theoretical 'idea of Man'—the philosophy and anthropology of any psychology—and the matter of 'what it hopes to achieve', which extends beyond an ontological question and engages with enquiring about the therapeutic direction of the treatment, ideas of normality and pathology and cure, we may think of this riddle of affirmation versus negativity differently. Whilst the ontological grounds between negativity and affirmation can be contrasted vividly, in the praxis, especially if we follow Freud, Lacan and Deleuze and Guattari from beginning to end, through their journeys, exploring potentialities of radical non-normative elements of their traditions, there is more opportunity of encounters, convergences and a possible thinking-with rather than a tired thinking-against. Neither Freud, Lacan nor Deleuze and Guattari were interested in maintaining paradigms of normality or corresponding with psychiatric dogma. In their own way, the singularity of their encounters in the clinic was their main compass. Psychoanalysis reinvents itself in each new session, yet, as Guattari argues in *Chaosmosis*, the "Freudian Unconscious has itself evolved in the course of its history: it has lost the seething richness and disquieting atheism of its origins and, in its structuralist version, has been recentered on the analysis of the self, its adaptation to society, and its conformity with a signifying order" (Guattari, 1995, p. 10). In this sense, holding on to the conceptual framework that anxiety is a vibration beyond the sheer subjective knotting that can act as indicator of possible new references or worlds adheres to the reality of repetitions and the possibilities of multiplicity in the clinic (Guattari & Rolnik, 2007). When asking what does psychoanalysis hope to achieve, the creative production of new possibilities of living is what brings together these theoretical and clinical approaches that have been thought-with each other and not just thought-against each other.

It is fundamental to acknowledge Lacan's rejection of 'adaptation'; and I see the project Deleuze and Guattari began—one carried further by feminist, post/decolonial thinkers and contemporary philosophers such as Suely Rolnik, Rosi Braidotti—as ethically attuned to the Lacanian spirit. At the end of the day, Lacan subverted mainstream psychoanalysis and revised his own understandings of it from the late 1930s until the late 1970s. When 'negativity' in its Hegelian sense is criticised by Braidotti (2011, 2019) or Deleuze and Guattari, what is being proposed is not an 'affirmative' version of psychoanalysis that is based on adaptability and the ego (thus a 'non-antagonistic' model as Žižek (2010) loves to point out in his rejection of Deleuzean ideas). Quite the contrary, the immanence of desire and an ethics of affirmation—when accounting for the unconscious, the realities of the clinic and suffering as well as for the modern humanist onto-epistemic foundations of Freud and Lacan—is a 'non-adaptability' of a constantly creative potency taken to its possible limits (Perci Schiavon, 2019).

Whilst repetition, suffering and a general sense of being stuck as well as paralysed by anxiety are often the reasons why people seek psychoanalysis—confirming the pull and gravity of the death drive—difference, production or affirmation lace the creativity of being, or the 'becomings' present in post-Deleuzean thinking. The creativity of living, the creativity of symptoms, the creativity of the enigmas of the body and, ultimately, the creativity to keep-on-living at times against many odds cannot but be witnesses to a plane of immanence, a desire that is production and affirmation that post-Deleuzian and Guattarian thinkers call 'Life' (Biehl & Locke, 2017). This juxtaposition of life and death, affirmation and negativity, critique and creativity, and the potency of engaging with this trouble is what I rescue in this formulation of anxiety, following the non-adaptability of the subject, the mistrust in the mirage of the ego and the Imaginary that are so fundamental to Lacanian psychoanalysis, but also keeping the 'Life Against Death'—to use Norman Brown's 1959 book title on Freud and Spinoza (Brown, 1959)—character of the affect of anxiety.

Freud's description of Eros and Thanatos, or the libidinal 'life' of affirmation and the repetitive, destructive Death Drive are paradoxes that follow his own complex journey of establishing a theory of the psyche with clinical preoccupations, cultural and political endeavours, and an 'ontologising' of suffering (one of his accomplishments but also pitfalls—Deleuze and Guattari (1983) view Freud's ontology as one of the neurotic European man, trapped in the Oedipal drama). For Freud, "only by the concurrent or mutually opposing action of the two primal instincts—Eros and the death-instinct—never by one or the other alone, can we explain the rich multiplicity of the phenomena of life" (Freud, 1937, p. 243). The Freudian writings on anxiety accompany his journey of making sense of this libidinal excess—of life, death, this beyond 'me'—as both connected to negativity and to affirmation. From his early letters to Fliess in the late nineteenth century, to the 1930s 'New Introductory Lectures', with his last theory of anxiety, this paradoxical version of the subject vis-à-vis libido, the body, affect and the conflict of the drives remains operative. Alenka Zupančič, arguing that both Deleuze and Lacan were in a sense very faithful to Freud's discovery, notices that "for both Lacan and Deleuze repetition is essentially related to the death drive as the fundamental matrix of the drive" (Zupančič, 2017, p. 166). Looking at Deleuze's writings in *Difference and Repetition*, from 1968, and comparing his reading of Freud's 'Beyond the Pleasure Principle' with that of Lacan, Zupančič (2017) also aligns them from the angle of an 'excess' that articulates or is articulated through repetition and one, as she reads it, that mobilises the affect of anxiety. She writes:

> Both Lacan and Deleuze insist that the excess (of excitation) does not exist somewhere independently of repetition, but only and precisely in repetition itself and through it. In other words, the thing in defence against which repetition mobilises anxiety exists only through the repetition itself. Repetition is to be found on both sides of this movement: repetition is what brings in the excess 'bound' by anxiety through repetition. The death drive already involves repetition, so that the repetition itself could be seen as split, or two-sided. (Zupančič, 2017, p. 167)

Anxiety situates the subject precisely in the failure of this repetition, the 'failure' or the mirage of the Imaginary-Symbolic knotting that we call the subject, which keeps the Real at bay. Anxiety, therefore, not only comes through in the defence against such excess as it is, even in strict Lacanian terms, an encounter with the Real, or an encounter with an excess. Lacan, in his radical project of re-reading Freud against the mirage of the ego, gives more emphasis to death, calling all drives a 'death drive'.[2]

[2] As Lacan writes in 'Position of the Unconscious', "Speaking subjects have the privilege of revealing the deadly meaning of this organ [the libido, which he is calling here an organ, naming it lamella], and thereby its relation to sexuality, This is because the signifier as such, whose first purpose is to

Whilst Lacan follows Hegel and Kojéve to the letter by assigning to negativity the condition of Being, it is in affirmation that one finds the possibilities of 'becomings', or of living and creating new repertoires of worlds, new Imaginaries that don't need to cross the structure of the Symbolic, rather, new Imaginaries that stem off the Real.[3] Guattari reverses Lacanian psychoanalysis from the logic of the Real (Sauvagnargues, 2016). Yet, still in Lacan, towards his later teachings, we can find if not open doors, at least some windows ajar for the possibilities of 'becoming'.

## Being and Becomings

Lacan's most complicated concepts such as the Real, the *objet a* and *jouissance* are wrapped in his theories of anxiety, leaving the possibilities of 'affirmation' hidden in the corner. Interestingly, towards his later teachings, when Lacan was working with what is known as the 'Borromean' Clinic or a Clinic of the Real, a Real that is no longer situated within the constraints of the Symbolic starts to appear. This later stage of his work, contradictory and complicated as all that preceded it, articulates the logic of 'Lack', which was the question of the Symbolic as not foundational to the subject anymore, whilst the body comes to the fore.

In some Lacanian psychoanalytic circles, an idea that "the speaking body is the 21st century unconscious" has been debated in recent years. This concept, or expression, 'speaking body', can be found in Lacan's later seminars and has been made popular especially after Jacques-Alain Miller referred to it in the speech and texts of the 2016 World Association of Psychoanalysis congress, that took place in Rio de Janeiro (Miller, 2014). The 'speaking body' is an elusive term that does not refer exactly to the fleshy body, nor to an imaginary body, rather, it points at a body through

bar the subject, has brought into him the meaning of death. (The letter kills, but we learn this from the letter itself.) This is why every drive is virtually a death drive" (Lacan, [1964]2006, p. 848). This deadliness is clearly attached to the signifier.

[3] According to Jacques-Alain Miller (2000) in 'The Six Paradigms of Jouissance', until seminar XX, Lacan emphasises language as the bearer of jouissance, but after this 1972–1973 seminar, jouissance gains some autonomy and a body that enjoys without language, without the Other, comes to the fore.

which the subject can come into being and, therefore, produce symptoms and a *sinthôme.* In this spirit, in the presentation of the *Scilicet* tome issued prior to this congress in Brazil, in October 2015, in which various interpretations and possible meanings of the term 'speaking body' can be found, an interesting definition of the potency of psychoanalysis is offered. It reads: "Psychoanalysis tends to make possible for each, according to one's singularity, the invention of an alliance between one's body and the resources of speech against the worst" (NLS, 2015). Whilst anxiety is not specifically reformulated by Lacan in his later teachings, considering his reformulation of the Real and the move beyond the Oedipal paradigm, there is scope for rethinking the Lacanian theory of anxiety through these 'vibrational moments'.[4]

The body, according to these late-Lacanian teachings, becomes an affective site in which the Real and possible new 'repertoires of worlds' (an expression I borrow from Rolnik, 2019) can be articulated. *Jouissance*, this ambiguous Lacanian term that is akin to Freud's libido but that translates from French as 'enjoyment', is central to such possible novel articulations. Miller (2000) has identified six different paradigms of *jouissance* throughout Lacan's teachings. The first ones still see *jouissance* as wrapped around language and the subject departing from language as such. The last of these paradigms appears in Seminar XX *Encore*, delivered between 1972 and 1973, where *jouissance* gains some autonomy, and from there onwards it is the *jouissance* of the living body that reorients the access to the Real—not the Symbolic, anymore—opening through *lalangue* the possibilities of an Imaginary. In the lesson on *jouissance* that opens *Encore*, Lacan says: "The habit loves the monk [alluding to a French idiom], as they are but one thereby. In other words, what lies under the habit, what we call the body, is perhaps but the remainder (*reste*) I call *object a*. What holds the image together is a remainder" (Lacan, 1998, p. 6). In this passage, the 'rest', or the excess from the subject's idea of oneself that is the 'body', is the anchor of the 'image'.

[4] After Seminar XI, Lacan mentions *angoisse* only briefly, once in Seminar XIII; once in Seminar XIV; once in Seminar XVI; twice in seminars XVII and XXII and for one final time in Seminar XXIV (15/03/1977). In the last definition Lacan characterises anxiety as '*symboliquement réel*'.

Miller (2001) writes in his essay 'Lacanian Biology' of a movement in Lacanian teachings that establishes the relation between body and language as one of satisfaction, signification and back to satisfaction—the *jouissance* of the signifier on the body beyond signification—in the later works. This movement is crucial to the matter of negativity and lack, as well as the riddle of affect and the body in and beyond Lacanian psychoanalysis. The question of signification, more specifically, led to the 'classic' Lacanian clinic, where interpretation was a principal tool of intervention. By shifting its focus away from meaning and towards the Real inscribed in the body, technique changes towards the 'cut' (stopping the session precisely when the unconscious stems off, protecting it from being wrapped by further Imaginary 'empty speech' once more in the session), or towards a skilled use of punctuation, where adding meanings (or stretching the Imaginary through the Symbolic) is substituted by producing, together, new verses, new poems that bridge this Real of the body into an inventive use of words—what I call a *co-poiesis*, inspired by Lygia Clark and Guattari. From Seminar XX onwards, the end of analysis changes path, once interpretations "by introducing more signifying material in the treatment, in fact encourage meaning-making by bringing yet more water to the mill of the unconscious. By contrast, the cut isolates *jouissance* in speech and prevents the proliferation of meaning that makes analysis interminable" (Voruz & Wolf, 2007, p. xi). In late Lacan, or from Seminar XX onwards, "Lacan downplays the Oedipus complex, seen as a mythical—and so imaginarised—version of unconscious organisation. And it is with the des-imaginarisation of the Oedipus that the deciphering of the unconscious becomes less central in the analytic treatment" (Voruz & Wolf, 2007, p. x).[5] Analysis, thus, becomes less of a matter of 'finding out' and adding meaning to a puzzle and more of a creative production of something else, of a new form of living, together. Through a rhythmic, poetic succession of constructions, a common ground is established. Again, analysis becomes a locus of *co-poiesis*, of sprouting new worlds. Here is the possibility for thinking and treating

[5] 'Des-imaginarisation' is a neologism connoting a draining of the Imaginary or of fantasy in the treatment. In practical terms, it means moving beyond an analysis of a family drama and towards the Real of the symptom.

'rupture' in the clinic differently—rather than inscribing it into predefined frames based on Oedipal identification, castration and domination, there is a communing, there is creativity in a creation of new ways of speaking, similarly to what Guattari (1998) proposed and what Lygia Clark realised in her practice.

In this shift towards the Real in Lacan's work, a similarity emerges with the 'affirmation', the multiplicity and the creativity that Deleuze and Guattari assign to a 'becoming'. With the move beyond Oedipus, beyond the Symbolic and the Phallic Law and beyond interpretation, "the relation to meaning and truth is less valued, and for the Lacan of the later period the analytic treatment is oriented on a reduction of the symptom. The *symptom* has to be emptied of the *jouissance* procured through its articulation with the fantasy so that the subject can make use of his *sinthôme* to love, work, and desire" (Voruz & Wolf, 2007, p. x). The symptom, which is what Miller (2001) rescues as a Lacanian 'biology', is the bodily, affective, excessive repetition, and to work through it in analysis, following such logic, is to find a poetic way out of the entrapments of such repetition that produces no difference into the horizon of difference and immanence.

Contemporary Lacanians, mostly the groups of psychoanalysts connected with the World Association of Psychoanalysis (vulgarly known as 'Millerians', which is not always a compliment), have been directing their studies, events and practice towards the later Lacanian teachings, where the Real and affects gain another dimension beyond the constraints of the Symbolic. The focus on the 'signifier' as cutting the body up and marking enjoyment/*jouissance* without any signification/meaning brings language back to its materiality. For Miller and contemporary Lacanians, the Borromean clinic was Lacan's attempt to formulate an Other for when there is no more Other, or what is the subject of the world like at the end of analysis (Chiesa, 2007). The Borromean knot was introduced in Lacan's teachings apropos of Joyce and his 'creative solution' in psychosis. Such theoretical interventions from the mid-1970s onwards see Lacan ceasing "to take his bearings solely from the differential clinic and introduces the perspective of the Borromean knots, with the consequent production of new statements on the symptom" (Brousse, 2007, p. 83). This means that thinking through the symptom solely through the differential diagnosis—the possibilities of structure of neurosis (hysteria, obsession and phobia), psychosis (paranoia, melancholia, schizophrenia) and perversion (sadism, masochism and fetishism)—crumbles, giving rise to a more 'singular' arrangement of the symptom.[6] As Marie-Hélène Brousse writes, "Lacan even reverts to an ancient spelling, that of '*sinthôme*,' to conceptualize what of the symptom cannot be reduced to structural determination" (Brousse, 2007, p. 83). The materiality of language, the Real of the symptom on the body and *jouissance* operate, as I argue, as indicators towards new 'becomings', where the Imaginary 'is the body' (Soler, 2014). Collete Soler (2014) writes about accessing such an Imaginary that does not rely on the structure of the Symbolic as a form of 'knowledge':

> In contrast with science, in psychoanalysis we are dealing with the horror of the knowledge at play, which, for everyone, is nothing other than knowledge—acquired with great difficulty—about his own unconscious, as real, and its consequences. Since Freud, the main consequence has a name: castration. This name is as suggestive as it is deceptive with its connotations of mutilation, which says—though not very well and invoking too much imaginary—that for the analysand this knowledge can only be approached at the price of passing through anxiety. (Soler, 2014, p. 204)

Going through anxiety opens the possibility of creatively forging one's *sinthôme*, or a new form of writing, speaking, dancing, a *poiesis* of Life. It is in this ambiguity of the affect of anxiety, which vacillates between 'being' and 'becomings'.

Whilst psychoanalysis—Freudian and Lacanian—is inscribed within an epistemological, ethical and scientific discourse of modern humanism

[6] In the late-1990s, Miller (1999) proposed the clinical diagnostic category of 'ordinary psychosis' to address exactly the modes of subjective arrangement produced after the 'fall of the Name-of-the-Father' (namely, the demise of traditional patriarchal culture). A polemic term adopted mostly by Miller's followers, it has also been dubbed 'untriggered' psychosis (Redmond, 2014). Whilst this is worth mentioning, I find the diagnosis of the 'end' of patriarchal culture very unsound and deeply Eurocentric and problematic. Also, the albeit nuanced pathologising of the end of the Name-of-the-Father is unimaginative. Following my Guattarian-feminist critique, I hold on to the clinic of the *sinthôme* via the method of *co-poiesis* and the focus on 'lines of flight'. Being so, the refused psychic alliance with Oedipus can be explored in the vibrational clinic of anxiety without necessarily subscribing to the differential clinic between psychoses, neuroses or ordinary psychosis.

(following Zaretsky, 2004; Foucault, 2008a, 2008b; Makari, 2008), it also destabilises philosophical and psychological/psychiatric assumptions and ideological dogmas about subjectivity, experience and suffering.[7] One of its most radical features is that it accounts for the subject and their symptom in singularity, with an unconscious activity that is enigmatic and irreducible. Another factor of its radical and non-ideological potential is that "it is a constant feature of the analytic clinic that it rapidly encounters the limits of its theoretical framework: a case of the real catching up" (Voruz & Wolf, 2007, p. vii). In this cartography, we locate the riddle of anxiety in the psychoanalytic clinic as situated between models of negativity and of affirmation in psychoanalytic, psychosocial and philosophical literature. This discussion was contextualised in the field of critical psychiatry and psychology, tacking the psychoanalytic usefulness to the clinic of anxiety. In order to address the 'estrangement' of the affect of anxiety in the dividualising dynamics of diagnosis and treatment of hegemonic practices in the field of psy through the last century, I asked whether psychoanalysis can bring anxiety from estrangement into entanglement. My answer is that it not only can but that it needs to.

## Aberrant Psychoanalysis

Thinking of the possibilities of ruptures and excesses within psychoanalysis, I propose to move beyond the realm of the abyss-within into the horizon-beyond. In doing so, I argue that anxiety (by being conceptualised as a vibration) must not be interpreted, rather it is to be worked through in the clinic by holding on to the situatedness of affective clues, identifying unconscious movements that collectivise and creatively travel beyond a structural and Oedipal circumscription of desire. This is the destiny of the Real, of rupture, that my creative clinic proposes; an

[7] La Barre, for instance, in a quite universalist and colonial tone argues that all anthropologists should read Freud and the classic texts of psychoanalysis once "the major premise of the analytically-astute anthropologist must necessarily be that nothing human can escape illumination from the penetrating, pan-human, and holistic psychology of Freud" (La Barre, 1958, p. 298).

aberrant psychoanalysis, a vibrational and urgent psycho-political intervention in the clinic.

Whereas the earlier Lacanian teachings focus on the process of subject formation as 'transindividual', or crossed by a shared Symbolic, organised by the Name-of-the-Father (his renaming of the psychologised and allegoric Oedipus), guaranteeing a cut that institutes desire as a lack, his later teachings will move away from such a structured engine. In Lacan's critique of the 'unitary' (or 'positive' instead of affirmative) subject of post-Freudian psychoanalysis, I have argued that it is not the Symbolic that extends beyond oneself, but the Real, a resisting excess that grants the subject a non-adaptive quality. Guattari's version of the Real encompasses affirmation rather than negativity or lack. The transcendent position of the Lacanian Law is put into context through the unveiling of its means of production.

*Poiesis* would come about for Guattari through possibilities of expression of ruptures, or, what is done to the Real (the *jouissance* of the Symptom, Anxiety, the Real of the body) in the clinical encounter. Is the Real compost for novel germinations or is it displaced in pre-existing narratives of a subjective drama? In other words, what do we do with anxiety—this appearance of the Real—in the clinic? Do we expand the possibilities of expression, supporting *poiesis*, or do we trim it with interpretations so that they fit into a pre-arranged composition?

According to Guattari, in *The Three Ecologies*, an 'a-signifying rupture' catalyses *poiesis* beyond the barriers of what the subject can grasp, or beyond our repertoire of worlds, as Suely Rolnik (2019) puts it. These ruptures need however to be offered a platform of expression. Psychopathological repetitions and anxiety are, for Guattari, rooted in the danger of such ruptures losing consistency and remaining passive to these moulds of repertoire of worlds (2000, p. 45). What Rolnik (2019) calls a 'repertoire of worlds', is an Imaginary-Symbolic arrangement that gets reproduced through pre-existing narratives, structures and psychoanalytic interpretation—the focus of Deleuze and Guattari's criticisms towards psychoanalysis. In his *Dialogues* with Claire Parnet, from 1977, Deleuze summarises his and Guattari's objections towards psychoanalysis in one sentence: "we only said two things against psychoanalysis: that it breaks up all productions of desire and crushes all formations of utterances" (Deleuze & Parnet, 1987, p. 77). Interpretations that fit or dissolve such ruptures, the Real, this excess, into a pre-existing Imaginary-Symbolic frame are, therefore, the counter-poietic element of psychoanalysis, according to them, neutralising, normalising, reducing or stopping any *poiesis* of new repertoires of the world, of situating the subject as part of a common of multiple others. Such interpretations operate instead by insisting on totalising universals that echo the humanist, modern, patriarchal and colonial roots of the Imaginary-Symbolic knot that situates psychoanalysis within an epistemology of a world in decline, or an 'anthropo-phallus-ego-logo-centric' [*antropo-falo-ego-logocêntrica*] (Rolnik, 2019) anchor of the capitalist colonial unconscious. Such a process has been called by Rolnik (2017) "the pimping of life".

Whilst I agree with Guattari and Deleuze in their critique of psychoanalysis, it sounds to me that they were talking to the most conservative side of psychoanalysis, omitting especially within Freudian and Lacanian teachings, the potentiality for a radical *poiesis*, or a practice of transformation.[8] I see it differently. To me, it is clear that in Lacan's later Seminars there is a shift away from the 'totality' of an Other, away from the Name-of-the-Father and away from structuralism.[9] The changes brought by his Borromean clinic or clinic of the Real address much of the critiques of Deleuze and Guattari: we find a clinic that works with punctuation and even some poetry, promoting the *sinthôme*. The *sinthôme* is poiesis.

My argument of 'anxiety as vibration' consists in first having mapped the vibrational possibilities in Freud and Lacan, taking in Guattari's eco-sophical ethico-aesthetic demands towards a possible co-poietic practice of psychoanalysis. In the affect of anxiety, an affective Real that extends

[8] Historically, in the 1970s both in France and Italy, psychoanalytic groups were set up by feminist collectives, deriving from Lacanian groups, such as the '*psychanalyse et politique*', of Antoinette Fouque, part of the women's liberation movement in France. In Italy, the *Gruppo Pratica Dell'Inconscio* also emerged with the necessity to speak, listen and work through the singularities within the women's movement that was so potent in Milan at that time. Psychoanalysis was seen as part of this liberation, allowing for a type of speaking and listening that would liberate colonised desires.

[9] This movement is more evident starting, for example, very clearly in Lessons 6, 7 & 8 of Seminar XVII, addressing 'Oedipus from myth to structure', and passing through the writings on sexual difference in Seminar XX, where we could see Lacan describing patriarchal universalism and idea of One-ness, and reaching his later topological attempts to wrap the Imaginary, the Symbolic and the Real in the body and the unconscious of the *parlêtre*, the speaking being.

beyond the subject and which is always in flux, produced at every encounter with humans and non-human forms, touches the limits of the Imaginary-Symbolic arrangement or of the repertoires of world that delineate the subject. This intensity, this excess, vibrates beyond the subject, calling for a germination of new worlds (Rolnik, 2019). Such an intensity is experienced as anxiety; it signals dangers to the subjective mirage, it dissolves Imaginary anchors, whilst it also pushes for things not to change. Anxiety vibrates the intensities of what is beyond the grasp of the subject, it destabilizes, overwhelms, paralyses. In analysis, the production of the *sinthôme*, when it is not self-referential but affective (or 'nomadic' in Braidotti's sense), is a provisional delineation of the subject, a new Imaginary-Symbolic knot that is pushed by the affective Real, lasting just long enough. The *co-poietic*, affective *sinthôme* lasts until it is subtly re-created in light of the intensities from the world in common. If the *sinthôme* is stiff, it will be no more than a neurotic symptom; if it is not there, life with others, creativity and connection are impossible. This 'aberrant' version of the *sinthôme* as *co-poietic* crystallises my formulation of anxiety as vibration.

## The Creative Clinic and Anxiety as Vibration

Psychoanalysis, at its best, is a practice of 'staying with troubles'. Conversely, at its worse, it is a practice that modulates collective horizons into an abyss within. The psychoanalytic landscape explored in this cartographic book entails developing a capacity of being able to stay with anxious troubles, crossing them, rather than brushing them off, resorting to quick-fixes. 'Working-through' in the treatment involves paying attention to symptoms, fantasies, excesses, repetitions but also possibilities, creativities and new arrangements that germinate in the analytic journey. In the case of the clinic of anxiety, in particular, moving from the edge of what gives consistency to the ego and exploring what 'gaining unconsciousness' (Tosquelles, 1991) can be like, without relying onto structural or Oedipally wrapped frames of interpretation, is the premise of creative clinic. In other words: *Wo Es War, Soll Ich Werden.* Where the vibrational unconscious is, there must I carry on becoming.

The unconscious, writes Lacan, in his very last seminar—Seminar XXV 'Le Moment de Conclure'—"it is that: it is the face of the Real—perhaps you have an idea, after having heard me numerous times, perhaps you have an idea of what I call the Real—it is the face of the Real of that in which one is entangled" (Lacan, January 10, 1978).[10] In this book, anxiety has been studied in and out of the clinic, considering its double-edge, as a paralysing and at the same time mobilising affect that exceeds a subjective delineation and its Symbolic-Imaginary anchors. Envisaging an alternative to what has been called the 'dividualising' politics of affect observed within hegemonic psy discourses and practices over the last century, an affirmative take on anxiety has been composed. In this book, but also in my clinical practice, I am inspired by Braidotti, Guattari and Rolnik, into committing to an eco-feminist approach, which means taking seriously the ethical demands of the twenty-first century (crossing feminist, decolonial, environmental, medical and epistemological debates) and the limits of psychoanalytic classic theories of Freud and Lacan when it comes to possibilities of an ethics of the Real, or of what extends beyond the subject. The challenge was to think about this excess characteristic of anxiety on the threshold of 'being' and 'becoming', not losing sight of the clinical application of psychoanalytic ideas.

Working with texts as puzzling archives, from Freud and Lacan, travelling through Lygia Clark and Deleuze and Guattari, the grounds and possibilities of affect have been unpacked. Affects (such as anxiety) are not reducible to Imaginary 'feelings', rather, encompass an ethical disposition to be produced by the affecting relations to others in a complex matrix that extends beyond (1) consciousness, (2) an Imaginary-Symbolic subjective delineation, (3) the Symbolic realm and (4) the binary of representation/non-representation and of sexual difference. By twisting the clinic of anxiety from the point of an affective Real, a subject of entanglement is welcomed into the couch.

Instead of insisting on a dividualising onto-epistemic frame of interpretation, a creative clinic of anxiety (one that does not 'dividualise')

[10] "*Et l'inconscient c'est ça, c'est la face de Réel… peut-être que vous avez une idée—après m'avoir entendu de nombreuses fois—peut-être que vous avez une idée de ce que j'appelle le Réel…c'est la face de Réel de ce dont on est empêtré*" (Lacan, January 10, 1958) in Lesson of 10th of January, 1978. Seminar XXV 'Le Moment de Conclure'.

operates as a platform for the production of relations, situatedness and a *sinthôme* that vibrates through such an eco-psycho-social matrix. By conceptualising anxiety as vibration, the possibility of a creative clinic unfolds. It is not just a matter of finding what anxiety is signalling, its cause; rather, what else can be constructed from such rupturing affect.

When encountering a patient or analysand suffering with anxiety, the expected path of the psychoanalytic treatment is to place this anxiety and what it is signalling as the compass for the direction of the treatment. As a compass, anxiety takes us to the edge of failed fantasy. In doing so, as we have navigated in this book, considering anxiety as a vibration adds a subtle and yet powerful ethical nuance to this direction. Instead of relying on interpretation, the function of identifications or of lack and castration; a technique of *co-poietic* constructions and punctuations will hold on to the 'lines of flight', or the 'creativity' in becoming that is the rhizomatic unconscious. Affective assemblage, rather than the dialectics of enunciation, anchors this approach to 'rupture'. Instead of gluing together shattered pieces into a wonky old piece, this approach entails assembling fragments into a new montage. Commoning, collectivising, situating, rather than individualising, privatising and universalising. What I have attempted to demonstrate is, to put it differently, the eco-feminist ethical impossibility of re/producing an estrangement of anxiety and the urgency of affective entanglement.

What Berardi (2018) calls the 'reactivation of the erotic body' through the tune of the vibrations of the world is what the direction of *co-poietic sinthôme* in the clinic can unfold. Anxiety is an affect, an affect that does not deceive, an encounter with the Real. As such, anxiety sits on the edge of being (as a signal) and possible 'becomings'—accordingly, operating as a theoretical and clinical riddle that re-orients Freudo-Lacanian psychoanalysis from a psychosocial perspective, acting, thus, between critique and creativity. What can anxiety do, and what can we, as clinicians, do with it? Anxiety is like a 'bird tapping on the window' (Guattari & Rolnik, 2007, p. 328) and the work of psychoanalysis is to find in these birds, and their wings, "indicators of new universes of references" (Guattari & Rolnik, 2007, p. 328)—or else, it will simply be a 'dividualising' practice.

## References


Berardi, F. (2018). *Breathing: Chaos and Poetry*. Semiotext(e).

Biehl, J., & Locke, P. (2017). *Unfinished: The Anthropology of Becoming*. Duke University Press.

Bradotti, R. (2019). *Posthuman Knowlegde*. Polity.

Braidotti, R. (2006a). *Transpositions: On Nomadic Ethics*. Polity Press.

Braidotti, R. (2006b). Affirming the Affirmative: On Nomadic Affectivity. *Rhizome*. Issue 11/12 (Fall 2005/Spring2006). [Online]. http://www.rhizomes.net/issue11/braidotti.html

Braidotti, R. (2011). *Nomadic Theory. The Portable Rosi Braidotti*. Columbia University Press.

Braidotti, R. (2013, June 19). Conversation with Rosi Braidotti. *nY.* [Online]. https://www.ny-web.be/artikels/conversation-rosi-braidotti/

Braidotti, R. (2017). *Per Una Politica Affermativa*. Mimesis Edizioni.

Brennan, T. (1989). *Between Feminism and Psychoanalysis*. Routledge.

Brousse, M. H. (2007). Hysteria and Sinthôme. In V. Voruz & B. Wolf (Eds.), *The Late Lacan, An Introduction*. State University of New York Press.

Brown, N. O. (1959). *Life Against Death: The Psychoanalytical Meaning of History*. Wesleyan University Press.

Chiesa, L. (2007). *Subjectivity and Otherness. A Philosophical Reading of Lacan*. The MIT Press.

David-Menard, M. (2014). *Deleuze e a psicanálise*. Civilização Brasileira.

Deleuze, G. (1992). Postscript on Societies of Control. *October, 59*, 3–7.

Deleuze, G. (1995). *Difference and Repetition*. Columbia University Press.

Deleuze, G., & Guattari, F. (1983). *Anti-Oedipus—Capitalism and Schizophrenia*. University of Minnesota Press.

Deleuze, G., & Parnet, C. (1987). *Dialogues*. Columbia University Press.

Dosse, F. (2010). *Gilles Deleuze & Félix Guattari: Intersecting Lives*. Columbia University Press.

Ettinger, B. (2019). Beyond the Death-Drive, beyond the Life-Drive: Being-toward-Birthing with Being-toward-Birth; Copoiesis and the Matrixial Eros—Metafeminist Notes. In P. De Assis & P. Giudici (Eds.), *Aberrant Nuptials: Deleuze and Artistic Research*. Leuven University Press.

Foucault, M. (2008a). *The Birth of Biopolitics: Lectures at The Collège de France 1978–79*. Palgrave Macmillan.

Foucault, M. (2008b). *Mental Illness and Psychology*. University of California Press.

Freud, S. (1925). Negation. In *The Standard Edition of the Complete Psychological Works of Sigmund Freud, Volume XIX (1923–1925): The Ego and the Id and Other Works* (pp. 233–240). The Hogarth Press and the Institute of Psychoanalysis.

Freud, S. (1937). Analysis Terminable and Interminable. In *The Standard Edition of the Complete Psychological Works of Sigmund Freud, Volume XXIII (1937–1939): Moses and Monotheism, An Outline of Psycho-Analysis and Other Works* (pp. 209–254). The Hogarth Press and the Institute of Psychoanalysis.

Frosh, S. (2006). *For and Against Psychoanalysis*. Routledge.

Guattari, F. (1989). *Schizoanalytic Cartographies*. Bloomsbury.

Guattari, F. (1995). *Chaosmosis. An Ethico-aesthetic Paradigm*. Indiana University Press.

Guattari, F. (1998). La "grille". *Chimères. Revue des schizoanalyses, 34*(Automne), 7–20.

Guattari, F. (2000). *The Three Ecologies*. The Athlone Press.

Guattari, F., & Rolnik, S. (2007). *Molecular Revolution in Brazil*. Semiotext(e).

Kojéve, A. (1969). *Introduction to the Reading of Hegel: Lectures on the Phenomenology of the Spirit*. Basic Books.

La Barre, W. (1958). The Influence of Freud on Anthropology. *American Imago, 15*(3 Fall), 275–328.

Lacan, J. (1964). Position of the Unconscious. In: *Écrits:* The First Complete Edition in English (2006) [B. Fink, Trans.]. W.W. Norton and Company

Lacan, J. (1976–1977). *Seminar XXIV, L'Insu que Sait de L'Une-Bévue S'Aile à Mourre* (1976–1977). [Online]. https://ecole-lacanienne.net/bibliolacan/stenotypies-version-j-l-et-non-j-l/

Lacan, J. (1978). Seminar XXV 'Le Moment de Conclure. [Online] https://www.valas.fr/Jacques-Lacan-Le-Moment-de-conclure-1977-1978-en-francais-et-espagnol,263?lang=fr

Lacan, J. (1998). *The Seminar of Jacques Lacan. Book XX: Encore. On Feminine Sexuality, The Limits of Knowledge. 1972–1973*. W.W. Norton &Company.

Makari, G. (2008). *Revolution in Mind: The Creation of Psychoanalysis*. HarperCollins.

Miller, J. A. (1999). *La Psychose ordinaire, La Convention d'Antibes*. Agalma-Seuil.

Miller, J. A. (2000). The Six Paradigms of Jouissance. *Lacanian Ink, 17*(2000), 10–47.

Miller, J. A. (2001). Lacanian Biology. *Lacanian Ink, 18*, 17–19.

Miller, J. A. (2014). The Unconscious and the Speaking Body. *World Association of Psychoanalysis*. [Online]. https://wapol.org/en/articulos/Template.asp?intTipoPagina=4&intPublicacion=13&intEdicion=9&intIdiomaPublicacion=2&intArticulo=2742&intIdiomaArticulo=2

Nedoh, B., & Zevnik, A. (2017). *Lacan and Deleuze- a Dis-junctive Synthesis*. Edinburgh University Press.

NLS. (2015). *Scilicet: The Speaking Body. On the Unconscious in the 21st Century*. Huysmans/New Lacanian School.

Perci Schiavon, J. (2019). *Pragmatismo Pulsional*. n-1.

Redmond, J. (2014). *Ordinary Psychosis and The Body: A Contemporary Lacanian Approach*. Palgrave Macmillan.

Rolnik, S. (2000, April 30). O corpo vibrátil de Lygia Clark. *Folha de Sao Paulo*, [Online]. https://www1.folha.uol.com.br/fsp/mais/fs3004200006.htm

Rolnik, S. (2017, November). The Spheres of Insurrection: Suggestions for Combating the Pimping of Life. *E-flux*. [Online]. https://www.e-flux.com/journal/86/163107/the-spheres-of-insurrection-suggestions-for-combating-the-pimping-of-life/

Rolnik, S. (2019). *Esferas da Insurreição: notas para uma vida não cafetinada*. n-1.

Rustin, M. (1995). Lacan, Klein and Politics: the Positive and Negative in Psychoanalytic Thought. In A. Elliott & S. Frosh (Eds.), *Psychoanalysis in Contexts*. Routledge.

Ruti, M. (2012). *The Singularity of Being: Lacan and the Immortal Within*. Fordham University Press.

Sauvagnargues, A. (2016). *Artmachines: Deleuze, Guattari, Simondon*. Edinburgh University Press.

Schuster, A. (2016). *The trouble with pleasure. Deleuze and Psychoanalysis*. The MIT Press.

Soler, C. (2014). *Lacanian Affects: The Function of Affect in Lacan's Work*. Routledge.

Tosquelles, F. (1991). Une politique de la folie. *Chimères. Revue des schizoanalyses, 13*(Automne), 66–81.

Van Haute, P. (2002). *Against Adaptation. Lacan's "Subversion" of the Subject. A Close Reading*. Other Press.

Voruz, V., & Wolf, B. (2007). *The Late Lacan, An Introduction*. State University of New York Press.

Zamboni, C. (2004). Al di qua di immanenza e trascendenza. Una via femminile all'essere. In *Annali di studi religiosi* (pp. 337–343). Edizioni Dehoniane.

Zaretsky, E. (2004). *Secrets of the Soul: A Social and Cultural History of Psychoanalysis*. Alfred A. Knopf.

Žižek, S. (2010). *Interrogating the Real*. Continuum.

Zupančič A. (2012, March). Not-Mother: On Freud's Verneinung. *E-flux*. [Online]. https://www.e-flux.com/journal/33/68292/not-mother-on-freud-s-verneinung/

Zupančič, A. (2017). The Death Drive. In B. Nedoh & A. Zevnik (Eds.), *Lacan and Deleuze- a Dis-junctive Synthesis*. Edinburgh University Press.

# Index[1]

A



B



[1] Note: Page numbers followed by 'n' refer to notes


A. C. Minozzo, *Anxiety as Vibration*, Studies in the Psychosocial,
https://doi.org/10.1007/978-3-031-62856-6

# GPSR Compliance

*The European Union's (EU) General Product Safety Regulation (GPSR) is a set of rules that requires consumer products to be safe and our obligations to ensure this.*

*If you have any concerns about our products, you can contact us on ProductSafety@springernature.com*

In case Publisher is established outside the EU, the EU authorized representative is:

Springer Nature Customer Service Center GmbH
Europaplatz 3
69115 Heidelberg, Germany

The manufacturer's authorised representative in the EU is Springer Nature Customer Service Centre GmbH, Europaplatz 3, 69115 Heidelberg, Germany. If you have any concerns regarding our products, please contact ProductSafety@springernature.com

Printed and bound by CPI Group (UK) Ltd, Croydon, CR0 4YY
01/10/2026
02225912-0004